SIGNS and SYMPTOMS of ATHLETIC INJURIES

SIGNS and SYMPTOMS of ATHLETIC INJURIES

James B. Gallaspy, M.Ed., A.T., C., LAT
Associate Professor
Curriculum Director of Athletic Training
The University of Southern Mississippi
Hattiesburg, Mississippi

J. Douglas May, M.A., A.T., C.
Athletic Trainer
The McCallie School
Chattanooga, Tennessee

with 280 illustrations

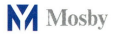

St. Louis Baltimore Boston Carlsbad Chicago Naples New York
Philadelphia Portland London Madrid Mexico City Singapore
Sydney Tokyo Toronto Wiesbaden

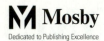
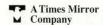

A Times Mirror
Company

Vice President and Publisher: James M. Smith
Senior Acquisitions Editor: Vicki Malinee
Developmental Editor: Catherine Schwent
Project Manager: Dana Peick
Production Editor: Cindy Deichmann
Electronic Production Coordinator: Peggy Hill
Manufacturing Supervisor: Karen Lewis
Designer: Amy Buxton

Printed in the United States of America
Composition by Mosby Electronic Production, St. Louis
Printing and binding by W.C. Brown

Mosby–Year Book, Inc.
11830 Westline Industrial Drive
St. Louis, Missouri 63146

International Standard Book Number 0-8151-4039-8

96 97 98 99 / 9 8 7 6 5 4 3 2 1

To my parents, who supported me when I made my choice of a profession; my students, past, present, and future; and most of all my family, Sue, Kim, and Jay, for their support throughout this project.

JBG

To my family, Cissy, Stacey, and Warner, for their encouragement, and my gratitude to my parents, for letting me become what I wanted to be.

JDM

PREFACE

Signs and Symptoms of Athletic Injuries is intended to assist the reader in the evaluation process of assessing athletic injuries and to help the reader make a knowledgeable decision for medical referral. Many textbooks give the signs and symptoms of injuries sustained by athletes; however, it is the intent of this textbook to also provide the reader with not only written signs and symptoms, but also illustrations of the injury. We realize that not all injuries can be illustrated, but for those injuries that can, by providing an illustration with an x-ray, MRI, bone scan, or other diagnostic image, the reader will be able to visualize the injury along with the signs and symptoms, thereby providing the teacher and student with a pedagogical aid to enhance the learning process. While this textbook is not intended to be all-inclusive, it is our intent to include all the injuries listed in the NATA Competencies.

Content and Organization

Section 1: Chapter 1 includes the definition of the terminology used through the textbook. Also found in Chapter 1 is a section on classification of athletic injuries that defines the different types of injuries the mechanism with signs and symptoms to help the reader classify the injury as first-degree, second-degree, or third-degree, and to decide if medical referral is required.

Section 2: Chapters 2 through 19 include injuries listed in the NATA Competencies that the entry-level athletic training student should have a knowledge of when sitting for the NATA-Board of Certification (BOC) Examination certification test. Each injury includes the **medical terminology** used to describe the injury/condition, then the **common terminology**, the **mechanism** of the injury/condition, the **symptoms** that the athlete would use to describe the injury/condition, the **signs** the athletic trainer would possibly see with the injury/condition, any **special test** used to evaluate the injury/condition, and the proper medical specialist that would be used for **medical referral**. Chapter 20 is a listing of common medical conditions written by a physician. Chapter 21 describes the general, immediate care of the athletic injury. A special test section at the end of each chapter describes how to properly perform any test selected to evaluate the injury/condition. When appropriate, we used plain film radiology, MRI, bone scan, or other diagnostic procedure that is elicited to diagnose an athletic injury/condition.

Section 3: The Appendix lists the different medical specialists used for medical referral.

After years of building on this idea, it is pleasing to be able to see one's concept take a solid shape and become what one thought it would be and to see this textbook become a reality.

It is our hope that *Signs and Symptoms of Athletic Injuries* will be an asset to both the entry-level athletic trainer and the certified athletic trainer, and that it will serve as a reference source for the evaluation and referral of the injured athlete.

ACKNOWLEDGMENTS

The preparation of *Signs and Symptoms of Athletic Injuries* was a collective effort of numerous individuals; many have contributed illustrations. This textbook is our way to recognize the many outstanding individuals in the athletic training profession who have helped make the profession what it is today and what it will be tomorrow.

Personally we would like to thank those students, past and present, enrolled in the Sports Medicine/Athletic Training Education Program at The University of Southern Mississippi, particularly Ms. Susi Soulie Folse; Dr. Doug Rouse of Southern Bone and Joint of Hattiesburg, Mississippi; Dr. Stephen Beam of Workwell of Methodist Hospital of Hattiesburg, Mississippi; Mr. Andy Bryan, A.T., C. and his staff at Mississippi Sports Medicine and Orthopaedic Center, Jackson, Mississippi; Mr. Ross Langston, Gulf Coast Orthopaedic Clinic; Dr. Frank Trundle, Jr., Team Dentist, U. T. Chattanooga; Dr. Kurt Chambless, Dr. Earl McElheney, and Dr. Scott Hodges of the Center for Orthopaedic and Sports Medicine, Chattanooga, Tennessee; and the nurses and x-ray technicians for their help and guidance with the collection of many of the illustrations. To the contributing authors, Dr. Stephen Beam and Mr. Greg Gardner, thank you for all your time and effort.

We would also like to thank the following reviewers for sharing their ideas and expertise:

Chris A. Gillespie, M.Ed.
Samford University,
Birmingham, Alabama

Colleen Keenan, M.S.
New Mexico State University,
Las Cruces, New Mexico

Charles Redmond, A.T., C., P.T.
Springfield College,
Springfield, Massachusetts

Catherine Schwent, our development editor at Mosby, has contributed many hours to the development of this textbook and we thank her for her time, encouragement, and most of all her patience.

CONTENTS

GENERAL TERMINOLOGY AND CLASSIFICATION OF INJURIES

Chapter 1

■ GENERAL TERMINOLOGY ■

abduction (ab-DUK-shun) Movement of a limb away from the midline of the body.

abrasion (a-BRA-zhun) A common wound in athletes, where the skin is scraped or rubbed away, exposing underlying tissue and capillaries.

active movement Movement of body part or joint through the range of motion without assistance.

adduction (ad-DUK-shun) Movement of a limb toward the midline of the body.

adenopathy (ad-e-NOP-e-thee) Swelling and morbid change in lymph nodes; glandular disease.

alkalosis (al-ka-LO-sis) Pathologic condition resulting from accumulation of base or loss of acid in the body.

aneurysm (AN-yur-izm) Localized abnormal dilation of a blood vessel, usually an artery.

ankylosis (ang-ki-LO-sis) Abnormal immobility and fixation of a joint caused by pathologic changes in the joint or its surrounding tissue.

anorexia (an-o-REK-see-a) Eating disorder; loss of appetite; aversion to food.

anoxia (an-OK-see-a) Lack of oxygen to the tissues.

apophysitis (a-pof-i-SY-tis) Inflammation of an apophysis, a bony outgrowth. Apophysitis usually occurs because of a tension force from a tendon, which sometimes leads to degeneration and fragmentation of the outgrowth.

arthritis (ar-THRY-tis) **(traumatic)** Disorder characterized by inflammation and degeneration of a joint; usually caused by repeated stress to the articulating surfaces. This stress causes the articular cartilage to slowly degenerate, while the surrounding bone and synovium thicken.

atrophy (AT-tro-fee) Wasting away of tissue or organ due to inactivity or neurologic problems; decrease in size and function of a muscle.

auscultation (aws-kul-TAY-shun) Process of listening for sounds produced in some body organs to aid in diagnosis and treatment.

avulsion (a-VUL-shun) An injury of the skin, muscle, or bone in which tissue is forcibly torn or ripped away from its source.

axonotmesis (aks-on-ot-MEE-sis) Nerve injury, second degree. Neurologic examination abnormal for at least two weeks; full recovery time varies from 4 to 6 weeks to 1 year.

bacterial (bak-TEER-ee-uhl) Pertaining to bacteria, microorganisms that cause infection and are not viruses or parasites.

bone necrosis (ne-KRO-sis) Death of a bone structure.

bone deviation (dee-vee-AY-shun) Departure of bone from normal shape.

bradycardia (brad-ee-KAR-dee-a) Slow heart rate.

bursa (BUR-sa) Small sac containing fluid; found in the fascia under skin, tendons, or muscles. Its purpose is to reduce friction between soft tissue structures and bone.

bursitis (bur-SY-tis) Inflammation of a bursa, a fluid-filled sac that facilitates motion and reduces friction. Most commonly a chronic injury caused by repeated trauma to the area surrounding the bursa; however, it can also be an acute injury caused by a direct blow.

cartilage (KAR-ti-lij) Dense connective tissue containing cells embedded in a ground substance or matrix; found at the ends of bones, within joints (*menisci*), and in the ear and nose.

cellulitis (sel-yu-LY-tis) Inflammation of cellular or connective tissue.

chondral (KON-dral) **fracture** Fracture to the articular cartilage at the joint. It usually is caused by a compressive or shearing force.

chondromalacia (kon-dro-mal-AY-shee-a) Softening of articular cartilage; it occurs most frequently on the posterior surface of the patella.

coma (KO-ma) State of unconsciousness from which a person cannot be aroused.

concussion (kon-KUSH-un) Brain trauma caused by the skull being jarred or shaken.

contrecoup (kon-tra-KOO) **injury** Trauma causing injury to opposite side.

contusion (kon-TOO-zhun) Bruise; an injury caused by a direct blow to the body resulting in capillary rupture, hemorrhage, and inflammation.

coryza (ko-RI-za) Cold in the head; an acute catarrhal inflammation of the nasal mucous membrane, causing profuse nasal discharge.

costochondral (kos-to-KON-dral) Pertaining to ribs and their cartilage.

costovertebral (kos-to-VER-te-bral) Pertaining to a rib and a vertebra.

cramp Painful spasm in a muscle.

crepitation (crep-i-TAY-shun) See *crepitus*.

crepitus (KREP-i-tus) Grating sound or sensation caused by the rubbing together of fractured bone ends (fragments), or swelling within a tendon (tenosynovitis).

dermatome (DER-ma-tome) Segmental skin area innervated by various spinal cord segments.

diaphoresis (dy-a-fo-REE-sis) Profuse sweating.

diaphysis (dy-AF-i-sis) Shaft of a long bone.

diarrhea (dy-a-REE-a) A frequent number of liquid bowel movements.

diplopia (dip-LO-pee-a) Double vision.

dislocation/luxation (luks-AY-shun) An actual displacement of contiguous surfaces of bones composing a joint; it is usually characterized by gross deformity and severe pain.

dyspareunia (dis-pa-RU-nee-a) Painful coitus.

dyspnea (disp-NEE-a) Difficulty with or labored breathing.

dysrhythmia (dis-RITH-mee-a) Irregular heartbeats.

dysuria (dis-YU-ree-a) Difficulty in urination, characterized by pain, burning, or itching.

ecchymosis (ek-i-MO-sis) Tissue discoloration due to extravasation of blood.

enthesitis (en-the-SY-tis) Inflammation at the attachment of a muscle or tendon to bone, characterized by inflammation, fibrosis, and calcification.

epicondylitis (ep-i-kon-di-LY-tis) Chronic inflammation of the epicondyle or the surrounding tissues, caused by a strain or contusion to the area, as in the epicondyle of the humerus.

epiphyseal (ep-i-FIZ-ee-al) **plate** Transverse cartilage plate near the end of a child's bone, responsible for growth of the bone.

epiphyseal plate injury Injury to the cartilaginous growth region in bone. It usually occurs in children between the ages of 7 and 16, because the bones at this time have not yet matured.

epiphysis (e-PIF-i-sis) Secondary bone-forming center; growth plate.

epiphysitis (e-pif-i-SY-tis) Inflammation of an epiphysis or the cartilage that separates it from the bone.

erythema (er-i-THEE-ma) Reddening of the skin.

exostosis (eks-os-TO-sis) Benign outgrowth of bone, usually capped by cartilage.

extension Motion of straightening a joint or moving the joint towards the dorsal surface of the body.

fasciitis (fas-ee-I-tis) Inflammation of fascia, a band of fibrous tissue.

fatigue Feeling of tiredness or weariness resulting from continued activity.

femoral (FEM-or-al) **canal** Opening in the abdominal wall through which various nerves, arteries, and veins pass to each leg.

fibroosteoma (fy-bro-os-tee-O-ma) Tumor containing bony or fibrous elements.

fibrosis (fy-BRO-sis) Abnormal formation of fibrous tissue.

fibrositis Inflammatory response causing an abnormal increase in the number of white fibrous tissue cells in the body.

flexion (FLEK-shun) Bending of a joint, which decreases the size of the angle.

fracture Disruption in the continuity of a bone.

groin area Depression between the thigh and trunk; inguinal area.

hematoma (hee-ma-TO-ma) Collection of effuse blood.

hematuria (he-ma-TUR-ee-a) Blood in the urine.

hemianopia (hem-ee-a-NOP-ee-a) Blindness for one half field of vision in one or both eyes.

hemoglobin (hee-mo-GLO-bin) Iron-containing pigment of the red blood cells; its function is to carry oxygen from the lungs to the tissue.

hemorrhage (HEM-e-rij) Bleeding; discharge of blood.

hypalgesia (hy-pal-JEE-zee-a) Lessened sensitivity to pain.

hyperextension (hy-per-eks-TEN-shun) Beyond normal extension, or straightening, of a limb or body part.

hypoxia (hy-POKS-ee-a) Low level of oxygen.

impingement Entrapment of tissue.

incision (in-SIZ-un) Open, smooth-edged wound caused by a sharp object or instrument.

inflammation Tissue reaction to injury or irritation, such as mechanical, pathogenic, thermal, or chemical. Heat, redness, swelling, and pain are indications of inflammation.

inguinal (ING-gwi-nal) **canal** Canal carrying the spermatic cord in the male and the round ligament in the female. It is 1½ inches (3.8 cm) long. A potential source of weakness; it may be the site of a hernia in the groin area.

intrathecal (in-tra-THEE-kal) Within the spinal canal; within a sheath.

ischemia (is-KEE-mee-a) Lacking blood; local or temporary anemia due to obstruction of blood flow to a body part.

joint Articulation; point of junction between two or more bones.

kyphosis (ky-FO-sis) Abnormal increased posterior convexity or rounding of the thoracic spine's curvature.

laceration (las-er-AY-shun) Wound with jagged and irregular edges, usually caused by a sharp or blunt object.

lateral Away from the midline of the body, pertaining to the side.

lesion (LEE-zhun) Injury or wound; a single infected patch in a skin disease.

lethargy (LETH-ar-jee) Condition of functional sluggishness; stupor; drowsiness.

ligament (LIG-a-ment) Band of flexible, tough connective tissue attaching the articular ends of the adjoining bones, serving to bind them together and to facilitate or limit motion.

lordosis (lor-DO-sis) Anterior concavities of the cervical and lumbar spine; this term also refers to an abnormal increased curvature of this area (swayback).

luxation (luks-AY-shun) Complete dislocation of a joint.

lymphadenitis (lim-fad-en-I-tis) Inflamed and swollen lymph glands, usually caused by a primary source of infection elsewhere in the body.

lymphadenopathy (lim-fad-e-NOP-a-thee) Disease of the lymph nodes.

lymphangiitis (lim-fan-jee-I-tis) **(acute)** Inflammation of lymphatic vessels resulting from the spread of infection through the lymphatic system. It is characterized by red streaks that are visible along the course of the vessels.

malaise (ma-LAYZ) Discomfort; uneasiness; indisposition; often indicative of infection or illness.

median nerve Nerve that controls sensation of the central palm, thumb, and first three fingers, as well as the ability to oppose the thumb to the little finger.

meningeal (men-IN-jee-al) **irritation** Irritation of the meninges (membranes investing the spinal cord and brain).

meningitis (men-in-JY-tis) Inflammation of the membranes of the spinal cord or brain.

menses (MEN-sees) Monthly flow of bloody fluid from the female uterine mucous membrane.

menstruation (men-stroo-AY-shun) Periodic bleeding from the vagina at approximately four-week intervals, in which the lining of the uterus is shed.

metaphysis (me-TAF-i-sis) Growing portion of a bone in young children; part of a long bone that lies between the diaphysis or shaft and the epiphysis.

metatarsalgia (met-a-tar-SAL-jee-a) Severe pain or cramp in the anterior portion of the metatarsal (usually the second and third metatarsal bones).

mild Pertaining to tissue damage, minimal damage of the structure.

minimal Least; the smallest possible.

moderate Pertaining to tissue damage, a partial tear in the structure.

Murphy's sign Sign of dislocation of the lunate bone in the wrist. The head of the third metacarpal moves proximally so that it is on the level with the adjoining knuckles and does not project distal to them.

muscle Tissue composed of contractile cells that effect movement.

myositis (my-o-SY-tis) Inflammation of a voluntary muscle and/or its surrounding tissue.

myositis ossificans (my-o-SY-tis aw-SI-fi-cans) Formation of bone or a bony substance within a muscle; it is usually caused by repeated irritation of an injured area.

necrosis (ne-KRO-sis) Death or destruction of tissue.

nerve Bundle or group of bundles of nerve fibers outside the central nervous system that connects the brain and spinal cord with various parts of the body.

neuritis (nyu-RY-tis) Inflammation of a nerve; symptoms associated with this problem can range from slight pain to paralysis.

neuroma (nyu-RO-ma) Tumor that emanates from nerve cells or nerve fibers.

neurotmesis (nyu-ro-ta-MEE-sis) Nerve injury with motor and sensory loss lasting at least one year, with no clinical improvement during this period.

osteochondral (os-tee-oh-KON-dral) **fracture** Fracture to both the cartilage and underlying bone within a joint.

osteochondritis (os-tee-oh-kon-DRY-tis) Inflammation of both the cartilage and underlying bone.

osteochondritis dissecans Fragmentation of cartilage and underlying bone, which eventually detach from the articular surface, creating loose bodies. The exact cause is unknown; however, it involves inadequate blood supply.

osteomyelitis (os-tee-o-my-el-I-tis) Inflammation and infection of bone caused by pyogenic (pus-forming) organisms; usually secondary to trauma to the bone or its surrounding tissue.

palmar (PAL-mar) Pertaining to the palm of the hand.

papule (PAP-yul) Red elevated area of the skin, solid and circumscribed.

paralysis (pa-RAL-ih-sis) Complete or partial loss of the ability to move.

paralysis, transient Temporary loss of ability to move; may be complete or partial.

paresthesia (par-es-THEE-zee-a) Abnormal sensation, such as numbness, tingling, or prickling, without objective cause; increased sensitivity.

passive movement Movement of a body part or joint through the range of motion by the athletic trainer.

passive stress Application of stress to a joint by the athletic trainer to test integrity of the ligamentous structures of the joint.

passive stretch Stretch of involved muscle or tendon performed by the athletic trainer.

periosteum (per-ee-OS-tee-um) Connective tissue membrane that covers bones, except at the ends.

periostitis (per-ee-os-TY-tis) Inflammation of the periosteum; can be chronic or acute.

photophobia (fo-to-FO-bee-a) Unusual intolerance to light.

polyuria (pol-ee-U-ree-a) Passage of a large volume of urine in a given period, as in diabetes.

pronation (pro-NAY-shun) Turning the palm of the hand backward or turning the foot outward.

puncture Piercing wound caused by a sharp pointed object.

pustule (PUS-tyul) Small elevation of the skin filled with lymph or pus.

radial (RAY-dee-al) **nerve** Nerve carrying sensation to the greater portion of the back of the hand; it controls extension of the hand at the wrist.

radiculitis (ra-dik-u-LY-tis) Inflammation of a spinal nerve root.

resistive movement Movement of body part or joint through the range of motion while the athletic trainer applies resistance.

retrograde amnesia Inability to recall events that occurred before a head injury.

sacroiliac (say-kro-ILL-ee-ak) **joint** Articulation of the sacrum and ilium.

scoliosis (sko-lee-O-sis) Abnormal lateral rotary deviation in the straight line of the spine.

severe Pertaining to tissue damage, a complete structure disruption.

shock State of collapse of the cardiovascular system causing a decrease in the oxygen supply to tissue; discrepancy between the cardiovascular system and its content.

silver-fork deformity Sign associated with Cole's fracture of the wrist, in which the hand appears as the curve on the back of a fork.

snowball crepitus Grating sensation on palpation of a tendon with tenosynovitis. It feels like small balls rolling up and down the tendon.

sprain Joint injury in which one or more ligaments are overstretched.

spasm Sudden, violent, involuntary contraction of a muscle or group of muscles.

spondylitis (spon-dil-I-tis) Inflammation of one or more vertebrae.

spondylo- (SPON-di-lo) Pertaining to a vertebra.

spondylosis (spon-di-LO-sis) Vertebral ankylosis (abnormal immobility and fixation of a joint due to pathologic changes in the joint).

spondylolysis (spon-di-LOL-i-sis) Breaking down of a vertebral structure.

stenosis (ste-NO-sis) Constriction or narrowing of a passage.

strain Trauma to the musculotendinous unit, usually from overstretching, forceful contraction, or predisposing fatigue of the musculature.

stress fracture Overuse, repetition of active movement causing an incomplete break in a bone.

subluxation (sub-luks-AY-shun) An incomplete displacement of contiguous surface of the bones composing a joint.

supination (soo-pin-NAY-shun) Turning the palm or foot upward.

syncope (SIN-ko-pee) Transient loss of consciousness due to inadequate blood flow to the brain; fainting.

synovitis (sin-o-VY-tis) Inflammation of a synovial membrane, a thin piece of connective tissue that helps reduce friction between bones.

tachycardia (tak-ee-KAR-dee-a) Abnormally fast heart rate; high pulse rate.

tachypnea (tak-ip-NEE-a) Abnormally rapid respiration.

tendon Tough, rope-like cords of fibrous tissue attaching skeletal muscle to bone.

tendinitis (ten-din-I-tis) Inflammation of a tendon; it usually develops from repeated microtrauma to the tendon itself or to the muscle-tendon attachments.

tenosynovitis (ten-oh-sin-oh-VY-tis) Inflammation of tubular synovial sheath surrounding a tendon.

testicle (TES-ti-kl) Male genital organ containing specialized cells that produce hormones and sperm.

theca (THEE-ka) Sheath or covering.

thecal (THEE-kal) Pertaining to a sheath.

tinnitus (tin-I-tus) Subjective ringing or tinkling sound in the ear.

trauma Wound or injury.

Trichomonas (trik-o-MO-nas) Genus of flagellate parasitic protozoa; *T. vaginalis*—vaginitis caused by a species of *Trichomonas* in secretions of the vagina.

ulcer Lesion on skin or mucous surface caused by superficial loss of tissue, usually with inflammation.

ulnar nerve Nerve that controls sensation over the fifth finger and lateral half of the fourth finger, dorsum and palmar surface.

unconsciousness Loss of consciousness.

valgus (VAL-gus) Force applied to a joint from the lateral side; angulation outward and away from the midline of the body. Could be a postural condition.

varus (VAY-rus) Force applied to a joint from the medial side; angulation inward and toward the midline of the body. Could be a postural condition.

vascular Pertaining to a blood vessel.

vesicle (VES-i-kl) Small sac or bladder containing fluid; small, blister-like elevation on the skin containing serous fluid.

virus Ultramicroscopic organism that does not have an enzyme system but parasitizes living cells.

volar Located on the same side as the palm of the hand or sole of the foot.

vomiting Disgorging stomach contents through the mouth.

■ CLASSIFICATION OF INJURIES ■
GENERAL SYMPTOMS AND SIGNS

Symptom is something that the athlete communicates (verbally) to the athletic trainer.

Sign is something that the athletic trainer can see or elicit through assessment procedures (facial expression of pain).

Loss of function is an inability to move the body part or joint through its normal range of motion.

Point to remember: Symptoms and signs increase with the severity of the injury.

■ CONTUSION

General symptoms Pain, loss of function, transitory paralysis, tenderness.

General signs Tenderness, ecchymosis, hematoma formation, inflammation, loss of function.

First-Degree Contusion

Mechanism Direct trauma

Symptoms Minimal pain, minimal loss of function, minimal transitory paralysis, minimal tenderness.

Signs Point tenderness, ecchymosis, inflammation, minimal loss of function

Second-Degree Contusion

Mechanism Direct trauma

Symptoms Moderate pain, moderate loss of function, moderate transitory paralysis, moderate tenderness.

Signs Point tenderness, ecchymosis, hematoma formation, inflammation, moderate loss of function.

Third-Degree Contusion

Mechanism Direct trauma

Symptoms Severe local pain, severe loss of function, severe transitory paralysis, severe tenderness.

Signs Direct and indirect tenderness, ecchymosis, hematoma formation, inflammation, severe loss of function, possible calcium formation.

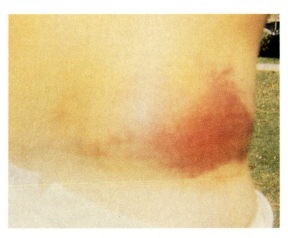

Contusion to the crest of the ilium (hip pointer).

▪ BURSITIS

General symptoms Pain, loss of function, tenderness.
General signs Redness, swelling, loss of function, possible calcium formation in chronic cases, tenderness, inflammation.

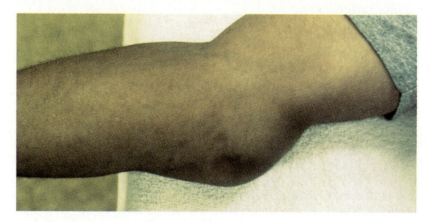

Olecranon bursitis in a football player as a result of falling on an artificial surface.

■ STRAIN

General symptoms Pain increased with active movement, pain on passive stretch, loss of function, possible snapping sound heard when injury occurs, muscle fatigue before injury, tenderness.

General signs Muscle spasm, swelling, ecchymosis, point tenderness, loss of function, loss of strength, hematoma formation, inflammation.

First-Degree Strain

Mechanism Minimal stretching or microtrauma to a musculotendinous unit due to excessive forcible contraction or stretching.

Symptoms Minimal local pain on active movement, minimal loss of function, minimal local pain on passive stretch, muscle fatigue, mild tenderness.

Signs Minimal muscle spasm, minimal loss of function, minimal swelling, minimal ecchymosis, local tenderness, minimal loss of strength.

Second-Degree Strain

Mechanism Partial tearing of tissue in the musculotendinous unit due to excessive forcible contraction or stretching.

Symptoms Moderate pain on active movement, moderate loss of function, moderate pain on passive stretch, muscle fatigue, moderate tenderness.

Signs Moderate muscle spasm, moderate loss of function, moderate swelling, local tenderness, moderate loss of strength, hematoma formation, inflammation.

Third-Degree Strain

Mechanism Complete tearing of part of the musculotendinous unit due to excessive forcible contraction or stretching.

Symptoms Severe loss of function, severe pain on active movement, possible snap or pop sound when injury occurs, muscle fatigue at time of injury, severe pain on passive stretch, severe tenderness.

Signs Severe loss of function, severe muscle spasm, inflammation, swelling, ecchymosis, local tenderness, severe loss of strength, hematoma formation with possible calcium formation, possible palpable defect in muscle.

■ TENDINITIS

General symptoms Pain on active movement, pain on passive stretch, loss of function, overuse activity.

General signs Swelling, loss of function, possible crepitus, possible calcium formation, inflammation.

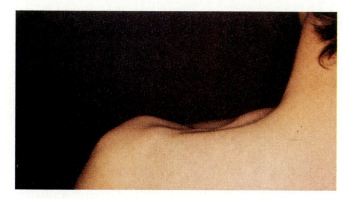

A clinical photograph showing localized swelling over the anterior aspect of the shoulder due to inflammation and effusion of the tendon sheath.

■ TENOSYNOVITIS

General symptoms Pain on active movement, pain on passive stretch, loss of function.

General signs Swelling, thickened tendon in chronic cases, snowball crepitus, inflammation.

■ SPRAIN

General symptoms Pain on active movement or passive stress, loss of function of the joint.

General signs Point tenderness at joint and ligament, joint instability with second- and third-degree sprain, swelling, hemorrhage, ecchymosis, inflammation.

First-Degree Sprain

Mechanism Minimal stretching of a ligament due to a direct or indirect force applied to a joint.

Symptoms Minimal pain on active movement or passive stress, minimal loss of joint function.

Signs Stable joint, tenderness at joint and ligament, no deformity, minimal swelling, minimal hemorrhage, minimal loss of joint function.

Second-Degree Sprain

Mechanism Partial tearing of a ligament due to a direct or indirect force applied to a joint.

Symptoms Moderate pain on active movement or passive stress, moderate loss of joint function.

Signs Ecchymosis, tenderness at joint and ligament, moderate loss of joint function, moderate swelling, local hemorrhage, slight instability possibly due to partial tearing of ligament, inflammation.

Third-Degree Sprain

Mechanism Complete tearing of a ligament due to direct or indirect force applied to a joint.

Symptoms Severe pain, severe loss of joint function.

Signs Tenderness at joint and ligament, severe loss of joint function, swelling, hemorrhage, ecchymosis, possible deformity, joint instability, inflammation.

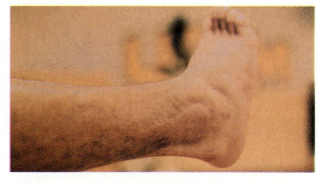

Inversion sprain of the ankle.

■ LUXATION

General Symptoms Pain, loss of function, possible numbness.

General signs Marked deformity, loss of joint function, swelling, point tenderness, possible neurological impairment.

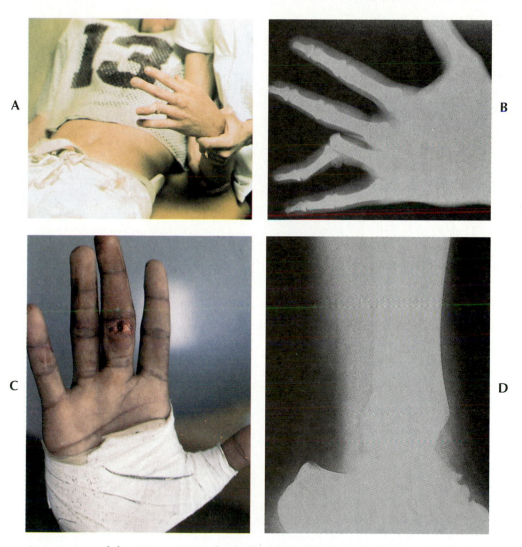

A, Luxation of the PIP joint in a football player. **B**, X-ray of a luxation of the PIP joint. **C**, Open luxation of the PIP joint in a football player. **D**, X-ray of a luxation of the ankle.

■ FRACTURE

General symptoms Sudden pain, loss of function, direct and indirect tenderness.

General signs Loss of function, possible deformity, rapid swelling, direct tenderness, indirect tenderness, possible bony deviations, possible crepitus, possible false motion, delayed discoloration.

■ EPIPHYSEAL PLATE INJURY

Type I Complete separation of epiphysis from the metaphysis with fracture of the bone.

Type II Separation of a small portion of the metaphysis and the growth plate.

Type III Fracture of the epiphysis.

Type IV Fracture of the epiphysis and the metaphysis.

Type V No displacement of epiphysis, but crushing force can damage growth plate, causing growth deformity.

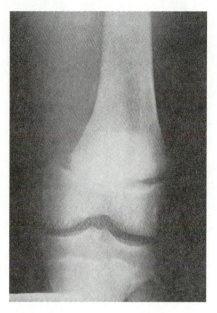

Epiphyseal fracture in an adolescent athlete at the distal femur (growth plate).

■ DEFINITION OF WOUNDS

Abrasion A rubbing away of a portion of the skin or mucous membrane due to an injury or mechanical means.

Laceration Wound or irregular tear of the skin.

Puncture Wound made by a pointed object.

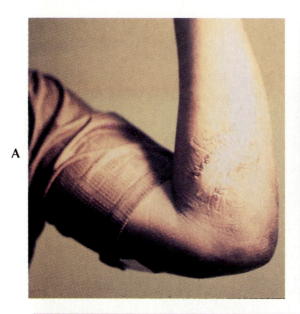
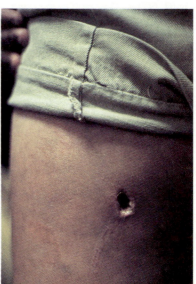
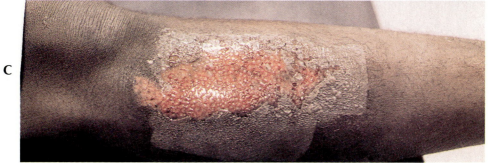

A, Laceration. **B**, Puncture. **C**, Abrasion.

HEAD INJURIES AND CONDITIONS

Chapter 2

Mild Cerebral Concussion
Moderate Concussion
Severe Concussion
Postconcussion Syndrome
Chronic Subdural Intracranial
   Hematoma
Epidural/Intracranial Hematoma

Intracerebral/Intracranial Hematoma
Subarachnoid Intracranial
   Hematoma
Acute Subdural Intracranial
   Hematoma
Skull Fracture
Migraine Headache

Medical Term	**Mild cerebral concussion**
Common Term	Concussion
Mechanisms	Direct or indirect trauma to the head.
Symptoms	Slight mental confusion; possibly some slight memory loss; mild tinnitus; mild dizziness; mild headache; pain in the area of the trauma.
Signs	Normal pupil reaction; normal balance; no loss of consciousness.
Special Tests	Level of consciousness; questions for memory test; pupil reaction test; check for positive Romberg's sign; cranial nerve assessment test; function test for return to activity.
Referral/ Diagnostic Procedure	Refer to physician if symptoms/signs persist.
Classification of Injury	Mild concussion

Medical Term	**Moderate concussion**
Common Term	Concussion
Mechanisms	Direct or indirect trauma to the head.
Symptoms	Momentary mental confusion; post traumatic memory loss; moderate tinnitus; moderate dizziness; moderate headache.
Signs	Normal pupil reaction; moderate balance disturbance; possible retrograde amnesia; possible nausea and vomiting; no longer than five minutes of unconsciousness.
Special Tests	Level of consciousness; questions for memory test; pupil reaction test; check for positive Romberg's sign; cranial nerve assessment test; function test for return to activity.
Referral/ Diagnostic Procedure	Refer to physician before returning to activity.
Classification of Injury	Moderate concussion

Medical Term	Severe concussion
Common Term	Concussion
Mechanisms	Direct or indirect trauma to the head.
Symptoms	Mental confusion lasting five minutes or more; severe tinnitus; severe dizziness; severe headache.
Signs	Abnormal pupil reaction; marked unsteadiness; prolonged retrograde amnesia and anterograde amnesia; unconsciousness lasting for five minutes or longer; possible increase in blood pressure and decrease in pulse rate.
Special Tests	Level of consciousness; questions for memory test; pupil reaction test; cranial nerve assessment test. Monitor pulse, blood pressure, and respiration.
Referral/ Diagnostic Procedure	Refer to a physician—medical emergency.
Classification of Injury	Severe concussion

Medical Term	**Postconcussion syndrome**
Common Term	Same as above
Mechanisms	Due to previous trauma to the head
Symptoms	Recurring headache; irritability; loss of concentration.
Signs	Irritability; loss of concentration.
Special Tests	Not applicable
Referral/ Diagnostic Procedure	Refer to a neurologist.
Classification of Injury	Not applicable

Medical Term	**Chronic subdural intracranial hematoma**
Common Term	Same as above
Mechanisms	Contrecoup injury, tearing veins that bridge the dura mater to the brain.
Symptoms	Increasing headaches daily.
Signs	Vomiting; behavior change; periodic drowsiness; post-concussion syndrome evident.
Special Tests	Perform a pupil reaction test; monitor pulse, blood pressure, and respiration.
Referral/ Diagnostic Procedure	Refer to a physician—medical emergency.
Classification of Injury	Not applicable

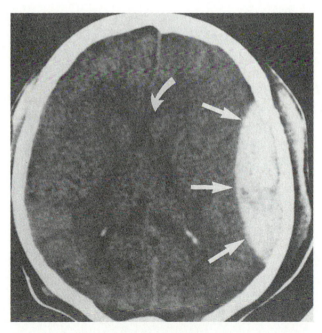

This enhanced CT scan shows a chronic subdural hematoma *(arrows)* that is causing a midline shift *(curved arrows)*.

Medical Term	**Epidural/intracranial hematoma**
Common Term	Same as above
Mechanisms	Direct or indirect trauma to the head, tearing the arteries in the dural membrane.
Symptoms	Headache
Signs	A short period of unconsciousness; some dizziness; vomiting; dilation of the pupil on the same side as the hematoma; muscle weakness on the side opposite the hematoma.
Special Tests	Perform a pupil reaction test; monitor pulse, blood pressure and respiration.
Referral/ Diagnostic Procedure	Refer to a physician—medical emergency.
Classification of Injury	Not applicable

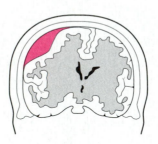

Shaded area shows where
epidural (above the dura)
bleeding occurs.

Medical Term	**Intracerebral/intracranial hematoma**
Common Term	Same as above
Mechanisms	A sudden, forceful impact to the skull causing blood vessel damage and hemorrhaging.
Symptoms	Headache
Signs	Rapid deterioration of neurological function; confusion; amnesia.
Special Tests	Perform a pupil reaction test; monitor pulse, blood pressure, and respiration.
Referral/ Diagnostic Procedure	Refer to a physician—medical emergency.
Classification of Injury	Not applicable

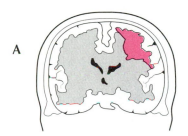 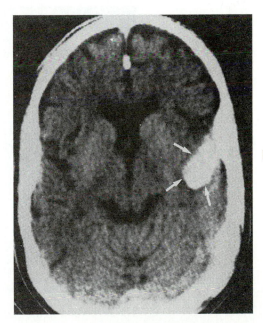

A, Shaded area shows where intracerebral (within the brain) bleeding occurs. **B**, CT scan showing a collection of blood *(arrows)* indicating an intracerebral hematoma.

Medical Term	**Subarachnoid intracranial hematoma**
Common Term	Same as above
Mechanisms	Sudden bleeding in the subarachnoid space due to aneurysm.
Symptoms	Severe headache, dizziness.
Signs	Syncope; vomiting; changes in pulse and respiration rates.
Special Tests	Perform a pupil reaction test; monitor pulse, blood pressure and respiration.
Referral/ Diagnostic Procedure	Refer to a physician.
Classification of Injury	Not applicable

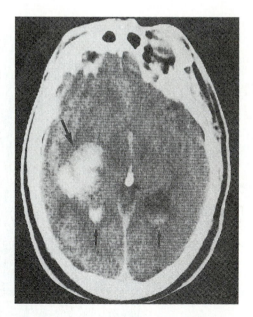

The arrows indicate a subarachnoid hematoma within the right temporo-parietal lobes and the posterior horns of the lateral ventricles.

Medical Term   **Acute subdural intracranial hematoma**

Common Term   Same as above

Mechanisms   Contrecoup injury tearing veins that bridge the dura mater to the brain.

Symptoms   Increasing headache.

Signs   Unconsciousness; dilated pupils on the affected side; diminished pulse rate; vomiting; dyspnea; increased blood pressure.

Special Tests   Perform pupil reaction test; monitor pulse and blood pressure.

Referral/ Diagnostic Procedure   Refer to a physician—medical emergency.

Classification of Injury   Not applicable

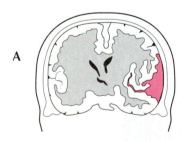
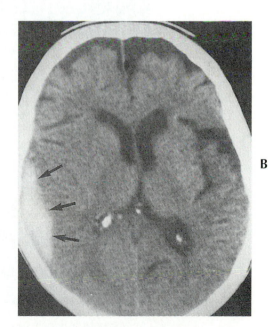

A, Shaded area shows where subdural (below the dura) bleeding occurs.
B, The arrows indicate an acute subdural hematoma on this CT scan.

Medical Term	**Skull fracture**
Common Term	Same as above
Mechanisms	Direct trauma to the head (skull).
Symptoms	Pain; headache; nausea and/or vomiting; memory loss.
Signs	Skull possibly depressed or deformed; abnormal pupil reaction possible; swelling; possible clear or bloody fluid running from the ear or nose; altered state of consciousness; bluish discoloration behind the ear called Battle sign, which may take up to 24 hours to develop.
Special Tests	Not applicable
Referral/ Diagnostic Procedure	Refer to a physician—medical emergency.
Classification of Injury	Not applicable

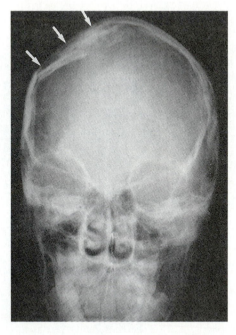

An x–ray of a depressed skull fracture *(arrows)*, following a blow to the head.

Medical Term	Migraine headache
Common Term	Same as above
Mechanisms	May be caused by repeated minor trauma to the head, possible vascular disorder, nutritional causes, or stress. All the causes of migraine headache are not fully known.
Symptoms	Hemianopia; seeing flashes of light; severe headache; paresthesia.
Signs	Nausea; vomiting.
Special Tests	Not applicable
Referral/ Diagnostic Procedure	Refer to a physician.
Classification of Injury	Not applicable

■ SPECIAL TEST FOR ASSESSMENT OF THE HEAD ■

■ CRANIAL NERVE ASSESSMENT

Name   Olfactory
Nerve   I
Function   Smell
Test   Have the athlete identity smell with each nostril.
Example: Gum

Name   Optic
Nerve   II
Function   Visual acuity and visual field
Test   *Visual acuity*
Have the athlete identify the number of fingers the athletic trainer is holding up or read something.
Visual field
The athletic trainer approaches the athlete's eye from the side.

Name   Oculomotor
Nerve   III
Function   Pupillary reaction
Test   Shine a light in the athlete's eye and compare pupil response to the light.

Name   Trochlear
Nerve   IV
Function   Eye movement
Test   Have the athlete follow your finger movement without moving their head.

Name   Trigeminal
Nerve   V
Function   Facial sensation, motor
Test   *Facial sensation*
Touch the athlete's face and have the athlete identify where you are touching.

Motor
The athlete holds the mouth open as the athletic trainer tries to close it.

Name	Abducens
Nerve	VI
Function	Lateral eye movement
Test	Have athlete follow athletic trainer's finger from left to right.

Name	Facial
Nerve	VII
Function	Motor, sensory
Test	*Motor* Request the athlete to smile, wrinkle their forehead, wink, and puff cheeks. *Sensory* Have the athlete identify taste.

Name	Acoustic
Nerve	VIII
Function	Hearing, balance
Test	*Hearing* Ask the athlete to identity a sound. *Balance* Perform a Romberg test, heel to knee test, walk, and finger to nose test.

Name	Glossopharyngeal
Nerve	IX
Function	Swallowing, voice
Test	Have the athlete say "ah," swallow, or test for gag reflex.

Name	Vagus
Nerve	X
Function	Gag reflex
Test	Nerve X is tested with nerve IX.

Name	Spinal
Nerve	XI
Function	Neck strength
Test	The athletic trainer applies resistance to a shoulder shrug and rotation of the head.

Name	Hypoglossal
Nerve	XII
Function	Tongue movement and strength
Test	The athletic trainer applies resistance to the movement of the tongue with a tongue blade.

■ TESTS FOR BALANCE ■

Romberg Test

The athlete stands with arms at the side, eyes closed, and feet together. The test is positive if the athlete falls to one side or sways back and forth.

Finger to Nose Test

Have the athlete touch a finger to the nose with increasing speed, with eyes closed. The test is positive if the athlete cannot touch the nose consistently.

Heel to Knee Test

Have the athlete move the heel of one leg to the knee of the other leg with increasing speed, with eyes closed. The test is positive if the athlete cannot touch the knee consistently.

FACIAL INJURIES AND CONDITIONS

Chapter 3

Tooth Abscess

Avulsed Tooth

Dental Caries

Tooth Fracture

Gingivitis

Intrusion of Tooth

Tooth/Teeth Luxation

Cornea Abrasion

Conjunctivitis

Eye Contusion

Corneal Laceration

Detached Retina

Foreign Body in the Eye

Hordeolum on the Eye

Hyphema

Impacted Cerumen

Epistaxis

Foreign Body in the Ear

Mandible Fracture

Maxilla Fracture

Zygomatic Fracture

Nasal Fracture

Orbit Fracture

Hematoma Auris

Lacerated Gingiva

Facial Laceration

Lip Laceration

Tongue Laceration

Temporomandibular Joint Luxation

Otitic Barotrauma

Otitis Externa

Otitis Media

Pericoronitis

Periodontitis

Periorbital Ecchymosis

Temporomandibular Dysfunction

Medical Term	**Tooth abscess**
Common Term	Bad tooth
Mechanisms	Decay into the nerve of the tooth; trauma; periodontal disease.
Symptoms	Severe pain. The tooth hurts more when heat is applied; the athlete feels relief when cold is applied; the athlete reports that it hurts to lie down.
Signs	Swelling of the gum near the tooth; the tooth may be loose; possible development of a fever.
Special Tests	Not applicable
Referral/ Diagnostic Procedure	Refer to a dentist.
Classification of Injury	Not applicable

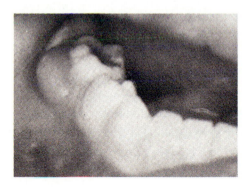

Abcessed second primary molar.

Medical Term	**Avulsed tooth**
Common Term	Extruded tooth; tooth knocked out
Mechanisms	Direct trauma to a tooth
Symptoms	Pain.
Signs	Tooth out of its socket; bleeding; possible lacerated gum.
Special Tests	Not applicable
Referral/ Diagnostic Procedure	Refer to a dentist with maxillofacial expertise. (Keep tooth in a moist environment—soak tooth in Hank's solution either in tooth socket or under tongue. Do not wrap in gauze.)
Classification of Injury	Not applicable

Medical Term	Dental caries
Common Term	Cavity
Mechanisms	Decay of teeth; disintegration of tooth enamel.
Symptoms	Pain, sensitivity to cold.
Signs	Tooth decay; possible inflammation; possible structural defect in a tooth.
Special Tests	Not applicable
Referral/ Diagnostic Procedure	Refer to a dentist.
Classification of Injury	Not applicable

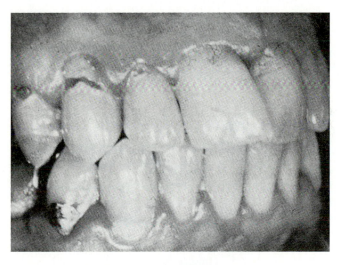

Rampant caries in a young adult.

Medical Term   Tooth fracture

Common Term   Broken tooth

Mechanisms   Trauma to a tooth.

Symptoms   Class I, sensitive from trauma; Class II, sensitive to elements; Class III, pain and bleeding; Class IV, severe pain and bleeding.

Signs   Class I, fracture in the enamel only; Class II, fracture into the dentin, with no pulpal involvement; Class III, fracture of the crown with pulpal involvement; Class IV, fracture of the root, seen with x–ray. Class II fractures may lead to abscess, depending on the amount of trauma. Class III and IV fractures will lead to abscesses.

Special Tests   Not applicable

Referral/ Diagnostic Procedure   Refer to a dentist.

Classification of Injury   See above signs and symptoms.

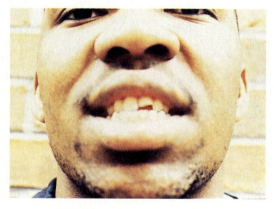

Tooth fracture caused when the athlete was hit in the mouth while wrestling.

Medical Term	Gingivitis
Common Term	Red gums
Mechanisms	Poor oral hygiene.
Symptoms	Bleeding of gums when teeth are brushed; discomfort.
Signs	Red, swollen gums that may bleed on probing.
Special Tests	Not applicable
Referral/ Diagnostic Procedure	Refer to a periodontist.
Classification of Injury	Not applicable

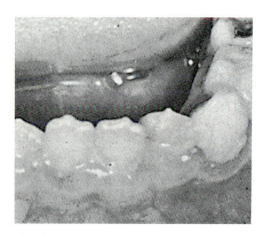

Gingival inflammation resulting from poor oral hygiene.

Medical Term	**Intrusion of tooth**
Common Term	Intrusion
Mechanisms	Trauma to a tooth, applied apically, that drives tooth into alveolus.
Symptoms	Tenderness and bleeding in the area; the tooth may be loose.
Signs	The tooth involved will be shorter than the others; possible bleeding.
Special Tests	Not applicable
Referral/ Diagnostic Procedure	Refer to a dentist.
Classification of Injury	Not applicable

Medical Term	**Tooth/teeth luxation**
Common Term	Tooth/teeth pushed back
Mechanisms	Trauma to the mouth, severe enough to loosen teeth.
Symptoms	Soreness and possible bleeding from the mouth.
Signs	Teeth loose; bleeding in the affected area. If nerve damage is severe enough, it will lead to abscesses.
Special Tests	Not applicable
Referral/ Diagnostic Procedure	Refer to a dentist.
Classification of Injury	Not applicable

Medical Term	**Cornea abrasion**
Common Term	Same as above
Mechanisms	A foreign object, such as a finger, in the eye scrapes or scratches the cornea of the eye.
Symptoms	Pain or a granular feeling in the eye; the sensation of a foreign body in the eye; photophobia; increased visual disturbances and decreased focusing.
Signs	Watering of the eye; spasm of orbicular muscle of the eye.
Special Tests	Not applicable
Referral/ Diagnostic Procedure	Refer to an ophthalmologist.
Classification of Injury	Not applicable

A 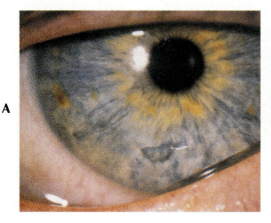 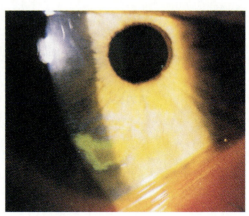 B

A, A corneal abrasion is hard to detect without staining the eye with fluorescein dye. **B,** After staining with fluorescein dye, the corneal abrasion becomes apparent as the green streak across the pupil.

Medical Term	Conjunctivitis
Common Term	Pink eye
Mechanisms	Infection
Symptoms	Irritation and burning in the eyes; visual impairment such as photophobia.
Signs	Inflammation of the conjunctiva, causing the eye to become bloodshot; swelling of the conjunctiva; in severe cases, sticky discharge from the eyes.
Special Tests	Not applicable
Referral/ Diagnostic Procedure	Refer to an ophthalmologist or a physician.
Classification of Injury	Not applicable

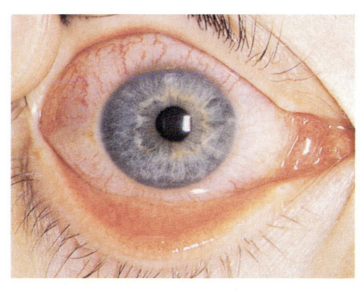

Infection of the conjunctiva results in the irritation of the eye shown here.

Medical Term	**Eye contusion**
Common Term	Bruise
Mechanisms	Blunt trauma, such as being hit in the eye with a tennis ball.
Symptoms	Pain; distorted vision.
Signs	Possible hemorrhage to anterior chamber; possible laceration; swelling around the eye globe; irritation; ecchymosis at orbit.
Special Tests	Light accommodation.
Referral/ Diagnostic Procedure	Refer to an ophthalmologist. Contusion to the eye can lead to several serious conditions, such as hyphema and detached retina.
Classification of Injury	Not applicable

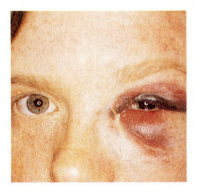

Swelling and inflammation due to direct trauma to the orbit.

Medical Term	**Corneal laceration**
Common Term	Same as above
Mechanisms	Trauma from a sharp object, such as a fingernail.
Symptoms	Pain in the eye; distorted vision.
Signs	Laceration of the cornea; the pupil may appear tear-shaped.
Special Tests	Not applicable
Referral/ Diagnostic Procedure	Refer to an ophthalmologist.
Classification of Injury	Not applicable

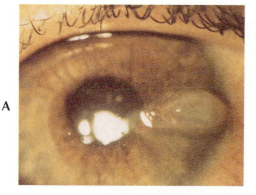 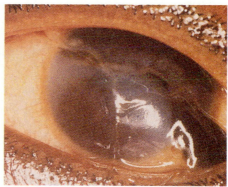

A   B

A, Eye perforation from a sharp object. **B**, Slipping out to the uvea from the inside of the eye due to perforation of the cornea.

Medical Term	Detached retina
Common Term	Same as above
Mechanisms	Blunt or penetrating trauma to the eye; common injury for boxers.
Symptoms	Blurred vision; the athlete sees flashes of light or floaters; athlete may experience a curtain or veil across their field of vision days or weeks after the trauma.
Signs	None
Special Tests	Visual acuity with each eye and compare.
Referral/ Diagnostic Procedure	Refer to an ophthalmologist.
Classification of Injury	Not applicable

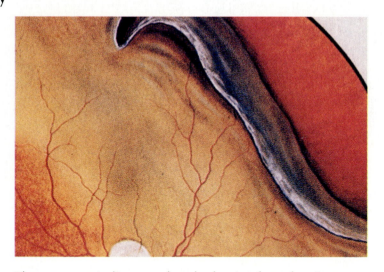

The gray area indicates a detached retina from the pigment epithelium, the posterior part of the retina *(red area in upper right-hand corner)*. Notice how the retina has fallen in this picture.

Medical Term	**Foreign body in the eye**
Common Term	Same as above
Mechanisms	Object induced into eye, such as grass.
Symptoms	Pain; disability; visual impairment.
Signs	Tearing of eye; excessive eye motion; spasm in muscles of eye.
Special Tests	Not applicable
Referral/ Diagnostic Procedure	Refer to an ophthalmologist if symptoms or signs persist.
Classification of Injury	Not applicable

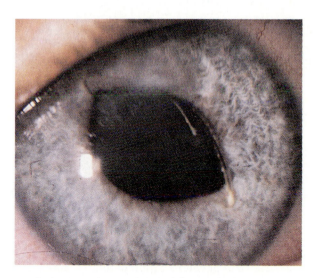

Eyelashes on the surface of the eyeball.

Medical Term	**Hordeolum on the eye**
Common Term	Sty
Mechanisms	Infection.
Symptoms	Pain; visual impairment.
Signs	Erythema; swelling; tenderness; boil-like lesion with a yellow center, usually at the base of the eyelashes.
Special Tests	Not applicable
Referral/ Diagnostic Procedure	Refer to an ophthalmologist or a physician.
Classification of Injury	Not applicable

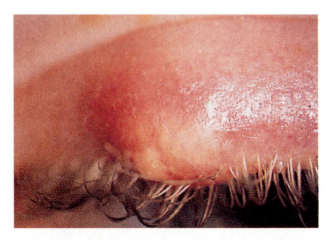

Swelling and inflammation of the sebaceous gland at the base of the eyelashes, indicating an acute staphylococcal abscess (sty).

Medical Term	**Hyphema**
Common Term	Same as above
Mechanisms	Direct trauma; blow with a blunt object.
Symptoms	Completely or partially impaired vision; pain increases with pressure.
Signs	Blood pooling in the anterior chamber of the eye; possible drowsiness.
Special Tests	Visual inspection with light.
Referral/ Diagnostic Procedure	Refer to an ophthalmologist.
Classification of Injury	Not applicable

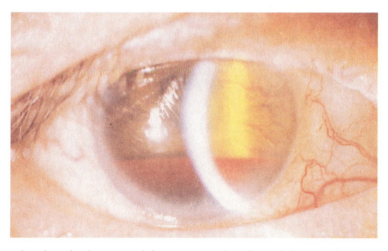

Blood in the bottom of the anterior chamber of the eye due to direct trauma to the eye.

Medical Term	**Impacted cerumen**
Common Term	Wax in ear
Mechanisms	Excessive wax in the external auditory canal
Symptoms	Loss of hearing; tinnitus; possible pain.
Signs	Dry, hard wax visible in the ear.
Special Tests	Not applicable
Referral/ Diagnostic Procedure	Refer to a physician.
Classification of Injury	Not applicable

Medical Term	Epistaxis
Common Term	Nosebleed
Mechanisms	Blow to the nose.
Symptoms	Pain; difficulty breathing through nose.
Signs	Bleeding; swelling.
Special Tests	Not applicable
Referral/ Diagnostic Procedure	Refer to a physician if bleeding persist. X–ray for possible fracture.
Classification of Injury	Not applicable

Medical Term	**Foreign body in the ear**
Common Term	Same as above
Mechanisms	The intrusion of an object in the ear, such as debris or an insect.
Symptoms	The sensation of having something in the ear; pain or discomfort; possible auditory impairment.
Signs	Pain or discomfort.
Special Tests	Not applicable
Referral/ Diagnostic Procedure	Refer to a physician for removal of the object.
Classification of Injury	Not applicable

Medical Term	Mandible fracture
Common Term	Broken jaw
Mechanisms	A blow to the side or front of the jaw.
Symptoms	The patient has pain opening and closing the mouth; malocclusion possible.
Signs	One or more teeth may be loose, raised above the plane of occlusion; there may be some bleeding. In the case of a complete fracture, some bone may be visible.
Special Tests	Not applicable
Referral/ Diagnostic Procedure	Refer to a dentist with maxillofacial expertise. X–ray should be done if a fractured mandible is suspected.
Classification of Injury	See Chapter 1 regarding fractures.

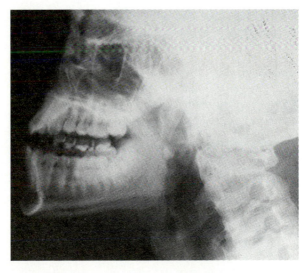

A lateral x-ray showing mandible fracture (notice the fracture line).

Medical Term	**Maxilla fracture**
Common Term	Same as above
Mechanisms	A blow to the maxilla.
Symptoms	Pain in areas; discomfort when patient tries to bite teeth together; tenderness to palpation.
Signs	Loose or displaced teeth; bleeding in areas; hematoma.
Special Tests	Not applicable
Referral/ Diagnostic Procedure	Refer to a dentist with maxillofacial expertise. X–ray should be done if a fractured maxilla is suspected.
Classification of Injury	See Chapter 1 regarding fracture.

Medical Term	**Zygomatic fracture**
Common Term	Cheekbone or tripod fracture
Mechanisms	Direct or blunt trauma to the cheek as in being hit with a bat or ball.
Symptoms	Sudden pain; direct or indirect tenderness; the athlete complains of pain when talking or chewing; the athlete will possibly complain of diplopia (double vision).
Signs	Depression deformity or possible prominence of the injured cheek when compared bilaterally by looking down over the forehead from behind the athlete; crepitus, direct and indirect tenderness; possible crepitus; possible epistaxis.
Special Tests	Not applicable.
Referral/ Diagnostic Procedure	Refer to a physician with maxillofacial expertise.
Classification of Injury	Not applicable.

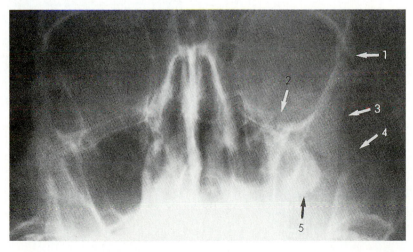

Waters view of left tripod fracture with comminuted body of zygoma demonstrating diastasis at the zygomaticomaxillary suture.

Medical Term	**Nasal fracture**
Common Term	Broken nose
Mechanisms	A direct blow to the nose.
Symptoms	Pain; difficulty breathing.
Signs	Bony deviation; possible crepitus; possible deformity; swelling; bleeding; direct or indirect tenderness.
Special Tests	Not applicable
Referral/ Diagnostic Procedure	Refer to an otorhinolaryngologist.
Classification of Injury	See Chapter 1 regarding fractures.

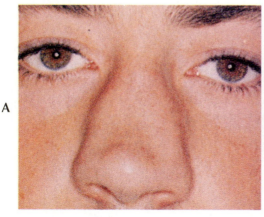 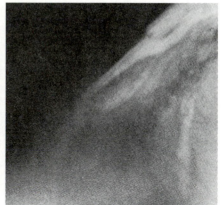

A, Nasal fracture indicated by bony deformity. **B**, X-ray of a nasal bone fracture.

Medical Term	Orbit fracture
Common Term	Blowout fracture
Mechanisms	Blunt trauma.
Symptoms	Pain; blurred vision.
Signs	Hemorrhage around the inferior margin of the eye; inability to elevate the eye; diplopia; ecchymosis.
Special Tests	Ask the athlete to look up, hold the nose, and blow.
Referral/ Diagnostic Procedure	Refer to an ophthalmologist.
Classification of Injury	See Chapter 1 regarding fractures.

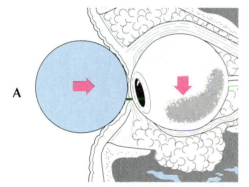 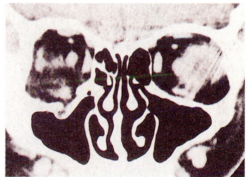

A, Mechanism of a blow-out fracture caused by the impact of a ball. **B**, CT scan of the orbit showing a blow-out fracture with disruption of the right orbital floor (left side of picture).

Medical Term	Hematoma auris
Common Term	Cauliflower ear
Mechanisms	Contusion or extreme frictional rubbing of the ear.
Symptoms	Pain or discomfort.
Signs	Swelling; puffy ear; formation of scar tissue resembling cauliflower.
Special Tests	Not applicable
Referral/ Diagnostic Procedure	Refer to an otorhinolaryngologist.
Classification of Injury	Not applicable

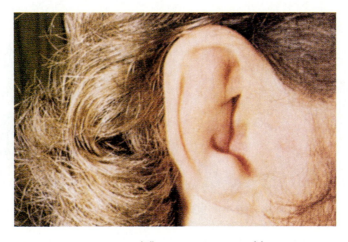

Hematoma auris (cauliflower ear), caused by separation of the overlying tissue from the cartilaginous plate, due to direct trauma to the ear, is often seen in boxers and wrestlers.

Medical Term	Lacerated gingiva
Common Term	Cut gum
Mechanisms	Trauma to the gums, such as a forceful blow to the face.
Symptoms	Pain, possibly severe.
Signs	Bleeding and soreness in affected area.
Special Tests	Not applicable
Referral/ Diagnostic Procedure	Refer to a dentist.
Classification of Injury	Not applicable

Medical Term	**Facial laceration**
Common Term	Cut on the face
Mechanisms	Tearing of tissue due to trauma.
Symptoms	Pain.
Signs	A jagged–edged cut to the face, with profuse bleeding.
Special Tests	Not applicable
Referral/ Diagnostic Procedure	Refer to a physician.
Classification of Injury	Not applicable

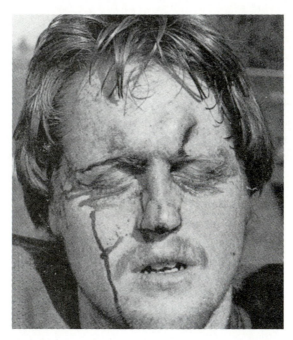

Facial bleeding after a laceration to the facial area.

Medical Term	Lip laceration
Common Term	Cut lip
Mechanisms	Tearing of tissue due to trauma.
Symptoms	Swelling and profuse bleeding due to the vascularization of the oral cavity.
Signs	A possibly jagged tear to the lip with swelling and profuse bleeding.
Special Tests	The athlete reports that it hurts to smile.
Referral/ Diagnostic Procedure	Refer to a physician.
Classification of Injury	Not applicable

Medical Term	**Tongue laceration**
Common Term	Cut tongue
Mechanisms	Tearing of tissue due to trauma; possible biting of the tongue.
Symptoms	Visible injury to the tongue; bleeding; pain.
Signs	Extensive bleeding from a cut or tear on the tongue. The tongue will bleed profusely because it is very vascular; therefore healing is also accelerated.
Special Tests	Not applicable
Referral/ Diagnostic Procedure	Refer to a physician.
Classification of Injury	Not applicable

Medical Term	**Temporomandibular joint luxation**
Common Term	Jaw is out of place
Mechanisms	Trauma, such a blow to chin.
Symptoms	Pain; malocclusion.
Signs	Malocclusion.
Special Tests	Not applicable
Referral/ Diagnostic Procedure	Refer to a dentist with maxillofacial expertise.
Classification of Injury	Not applicable

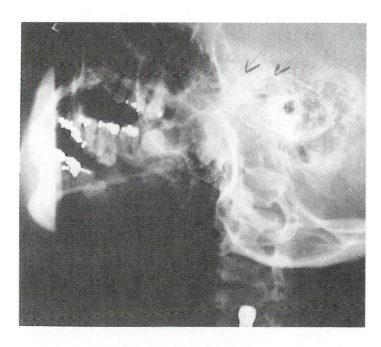

Dislocation of the jaw (right temporomandibular joint).

Medical Term	**Otitic barotrauma**
Common Term	Pressure injury
Mechanisms	Lack of pressure equalization, possibly due to cold, allergy, or infection. This is a common injury in diving, scuba diving, parachuting, and sports flying.
Symptoms	Increased pressure in ear; possible pain, hearing impairment.
Signs	Possible middle ear hemorrhage; possible bursting of ear drum.
Special Tests	Not applicable
Referral/ Diagnostic Procedure	Refer to an otorhinolaryngologist.
Classification of Injury	Not applicable

Medical Term	**Otitis externa**
Common Term	Swimmer's ear
Mechanisms	Development of bacteria from water in ear.
Symptoms	Itching; pain; possible hearing loss.
Signs	Possible discharge from the ear; pain produced by pulling downward on ear lobe.
Special Tests	Not applicable
Referral/ Diagnostic Procedure	Refer to an otorhinolaryngologist or a physician.
Classification of Injury	Not applicable

Medical Term	Otitis media
Common Term	Infected ear
Mechanisms	Infection or trauma to the tympanic membrane.
Symptoms	Severe earache; possible hearing loss.
Signs	Possible nausea and vomiting; red ear drum.
Special Tests	Not applicable
Referral/ Diagnostic Procedure	Refer to an otorhinolaryngologist.
Classification of Injury	Not applicable

Medical Term	Pericoronitis
Common Term	Swelling over teeth
Mechanisms	Infection and inflammation of the gingiva next to unerupted tooth.
Symptoms	Pain and swelling of the gums in one area; a bad taste in the mouth; bad breath; possibly an earache. Inflammation makes it hurt to brush the teeth in this area, so the patient does not, and this complicates the process.
Signs	Swollen gingiva over an unerupted tooth.
Special Tests	Not applicable
Referral/ Diagnostic Procedure	Refer to a periodontist.
Classification of Injury	Not applicable

Medical Term	**Periodontitis**
Common Term	Pyorrhea
Mechanisms	Severe inflammation of gingival tissue due to lack of oral hygiene, which allows bacteria to proliferate in the tissue.
Symptoms	Teeth that hurt and are loose; bleeding; bad breath odor; sensitivity of the roots of the teeth due to bone loss.
Signs	Bleeding gums; tartar buildup; bad breath odor.
Special Tests	Not applicable
Referral/ Diagnostic Procedure	Refer to a periodontist.
Classification of Injury	Not applicable

Medical Term	**Periorbital ecchymosis**
Common Term	Black eye
Mechanisms	Blunt injury to the periorbital region.
Symptoms	Pain and visual impairment.
Signs	Swelling; ecchymosis; restriction of lid movement.
Special Tests	Not applicable
Referral/ Diagnostic Procedure	Refer to an ophthalmologist.
Classification of Injury	Not applicable

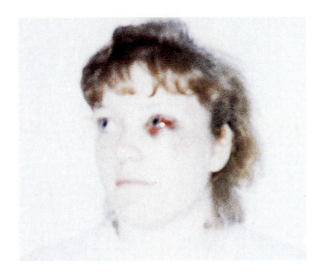

Periorbital ecchymosis (black eye) secondary to an eye contusion from direct trauma to the eye or orbit.

Medical Term	**Temporomandibular dysfunction**
Common Term	TMJ dysfunction
Mechanisms	Improper alignment of teeth in occlusion; grinding of teeth at night; trauma; rheumatic fever.
Symptoms	Crepitus in the joint of the jaw; pain in the head (headache), neck, and jaw anterior to ear.
Signs	Mouth can open or close, but teeth will not meet when closed; pain is persistent.
Special Tests	Not applicable
Referral/ Diagnostic Procedure	Refer to a dentist with maxillofacial expertise.
Classification of Injury	Not applicable

Neck Injuries and Conditions

Chapter 4

Medical Term	**Brachial plexus axonotmesis**
Common Term	Burner/stinger
Mechanisms	Forced lateral flexion of the neck with the opposite shoulder depressed; hyperextension of the neck; lateral flexion to the side of the injury.
Symptoms	Pain in the shoulder, arm, and hand; numbness or tingling in the shoulder, arm, and hand; tenderness over the brachial plexus–clavicular area; tenderness over the upper middle portion of the trapezius muscle.
Signs	Athlete holds the arm to the side with the shoulder depressed; muscle weakness; loss of function; loss of sensation over more than one dermatome; abnormal results on neurological examination for at least two weeks. Full recovery varies from 4 to 6 weeks to a year.
Special Tests	Brachial plexus evaluation test.
Referral/ Diagnostic Procedure	Refer to a neurologist.
Classification of Injury	Not applicable

Medical Term	**Brachial plexus neuropraxia**
Common Term	Pinched nerve/burner/stinger
Mechanisms	Neck forced into lateral flexion with the opposite shoulder depressed; hyperextension of the neck; lateral flexion to the side of the injury.
Symptoms	Pain in the shoulder, arm, and hand; numbness and tingling in the shoulder, arm, and hand; tenderness over the brachial plexus–clavicular area; tenderness over the upper middle position of the trapezius muscle.
Signs	Athlete holds the arm to the side with the shoulder depressed. Signs include loss of function; loss of sensation over more than one dermatome; numbness may last minutes to hours; complete recovery usually occurs in two weeks.
Special Tests	Brachial plexus evaluation test.
Referral/ Diagnostic Procedure	Refer to a neurologist.
Classification of Injury	Not applicable

Medical Term	Brachial plexus neurotomesis
Common Term	Burner/stinger
Mechanisms	Neck forced into lateral flexion with the opposite shoulder depressed; hyperextension of the neck; lateral flexion to the side of the injury.
Symptoms	Pain in the shoulder, arm, and hand; numbness and tingling in the shoulder, arm, and hand; tenderness over the brachial plexus–clavicular area; tenderness over the upper middle portion of the trapezius muscle.
Signs	The athlete holds the arm to the side with the shoulder depressed. Signs include muscle weakness, loss of function, and loss of sensation over more than one dermatome; motor and sensory loss for at least one year in duration with no clinical improvement during this period.
Special Tests	Brachial plexus evaluation test.
Referral/ Diagnostic Procedure	Refer to a neurologist.
Classification of Injury	Not applicable

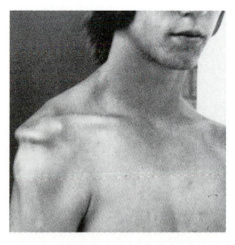

Atrophy of the deltoid muscle due to repeated brachial plexus trauma.

Medical Term   Throat/larynx contusion

Common Term   Clothesline injury

Mechanisms   Direct trauma to the anterior portion of the neck.

Symptoms   Pain in the throat area and problems swallowing; tenderness; dyspnea.

Signs   Swelling; spasmodic coughing; hoarse voice; direct tenderness; hemoptysis (expectoration of blood); being unable to breath normally may indicate a possible fracture to the throat cartilage.

Special Tests   Not applicable

Referral/   Refer to an otorhinolaryngologist.
Diagnostic
Procedure

Classification   Not applicable
of Injury

Medical Term	**Larynx fracture**
Common Term	Same as above
Mechanisms	Direct trauma to the airway.
Symptoms	Pain in the throat area; pain on swallowing; dyspnea.
Signs	Swelling and crepitus of the anterior neck; possible respiratory distress; obliteration of normal cartilaginous landmarks of the anterior throat; coughing up of frothy blood.
Special Tests	Not applicable
Referral/ Diagnostic Procedure	Refer to an otorhinolaryngologist.
Classification of Injury	Not applicable

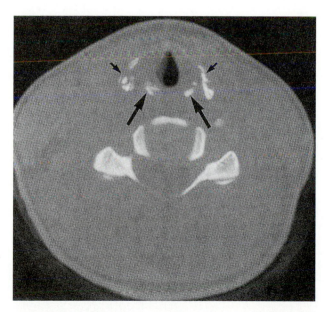

Fractures of the thyroid cartilage *(small arrows)* and cricoid cartilage *(large arrows)* on a CT scan.

Medical Term	**Cervical vertebra fracture**
Common Term	Broken neck
Mechanisms	Axial loading; trauma from multidirectional forces.
Symptoms	Sudden pain in the neck, shoulder and arm; direct and indirect tenderness; tingling, possible numbness; loss of neck function.
Signs	Loss of neck function; possible deformity paraspinous muscle spasm; possible loss of sensory function; possible loss of reflexes; possible tingling pain over vertebrae at the site of the fracture.
Special Tests	Reflex test; sensory test.
Referral/ Diagnostic Procedure	Refer to a orthopedic surgeon—medical emergency. (Stabilize head and neck before transporting the athlete.) X–ray.
Classification of Injury	Not applicable

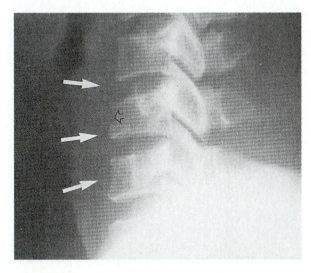

Anterior "tear drop" fracture at C5 due to a diving injury, with posterior movement of the vertebral body into the spinal canal. *Arrows* indicate a widening of the facet joints.

Medical Term	**Intervertebral disc rupture/cervical herniation**
Common Term	Slipped disc/ruptured disc
Mechanisms	Compressive loading.
Symptoms	Severe pain in the neck, shoulder, and arm; associated numbness, tingling where there is muscle weakness; increased pain when coughing or sneezing.
Signs	Compression pressure on the head with the neck extended and lateral bend to the involved side reproduces the pain; possible motor weakness of the wrist and finger extensors and flexors; possible sensory loss, possible loss of triceps and biceps reflexes.
Special Tests	Distraction test; compression test; Valsalva test.
Referral/ Diagnostic Procedure	Refer to a neurosurgeon.
Classification of Injury	Not applicable

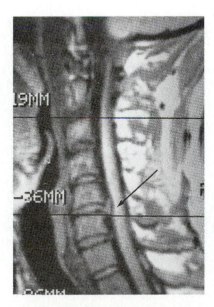

C5–C6 cervical disk herniation
on MRI (arrow).

Medical Term	**Cervical vertebrae luxation**
Common Term	Dislocated vertebrae
Mechanisms	Axial loading; moderate force with flexion and rotation of the head.
Symptoms	Sudden pain in the neck, shoulder, and arm. Direct and indirect tenderness in the neck; tingling; numbness or loss of neck movement.
Signs	Deformity (may not be visible); paraspinal muscle spasm; possible loss of sensory function; possible loss of reflexes; weakness of the upper extremity with nerve root involvement; possible quadriplegia.
Special Tests	Not applicable
Referral/ Diagnostic Procedure	Refer to a neurosurgeon—medical emergency. (Stabilize head and neck before transporting the athlete.)
Classification of Injury	Not applicable

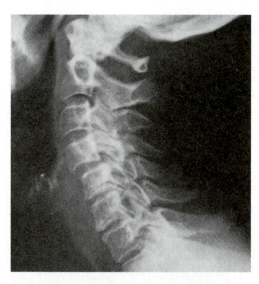

Lateral x–ray demonstrating a cervical vertebral luxation at C4–C5 from a riding accident.

Medical Term	**Nerve root compression**
Common Term	Contusion of nerve
Mechanisms	Indirect trauma; lateral flexion of the neck as in a brachial plexus injury.
Symptoms	Numbness; paresthesia; hyperflexion or lateral flexion of the neck on the same side as the symptoms may cause pain and/or numbness.
Signs	Tenderness over posterior aspect of the neck; decreased sensation in one or more definable dermatomes; muscle weakness; pain on downward pressure of the head with the chin in the supraclavicular fossa on the same side as the injury; decreased reflexes.
Special Tests	Distraction test; compression test; Valsalva test; range of motion movements.
Referral/ Diagnostic Procedure	Refer to a neurologist or a neurosurgeon.
Classification of Injury	Not applicable

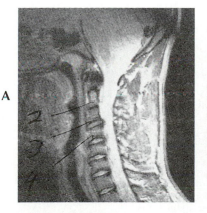 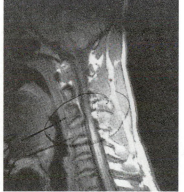

A   B

Herniated cervical disk indicated with myelogram (**A**) and CT scan (**B**) causing nerve root compression at the C3–C4 level in flexion.

Medical Term	**Spinal cord injury/concussion**
Common Term	Transient quadriplegia
Mechanisms	Indirect trauma, as in axial loading to the cervical spine; indirect trauma to the skull or face.
Symptoms	Immediate, transient loss of neurologic function including motor weakness and loss of sensation; loss of bladder and bowel function.
Signs	Transient paralysis with recovery; loss of normal reflexes and presence of pathologic reflexes; loss in sensory sensation below the level of injury; possible decrease in blood pressure; possible decrease in respiration.
Special Tests	Test for neurologic sensations.
Referral/ Diagnostic Procedure	Refer to a neurosurgeon—medical emergency.
Classification of Injury	Not applicable

Medical Term	**Spinal cord injury/contusion**
Common Term	Same as above
Mechanisms	Axial loading to the cervical spine with associated swelling of the spinal cord; indirect trauma to the skull or face.
Symptoms	Immediate loss of neurologic function including motor weakness and loss of sensation; bladder and bowel dysfunction.
Signs	Partial or permanent impairment of neurologic function; loss of normal reflexes and presence of pathologic reflexes; partial paralysis or total paralysis of extremities and trunk.
Special Tests	Test for neurologic sensations.
Referral/ Diagnostic Procedure	Refer to a neurosurgeon—medical emergency.
Classification of Injury	Not applicable

Medical Term	Cervical sprain
Common Term	Whiplash injury
Mechanisms	Forced hyperextension or hyperflexion or abnormal range of motion of the neck; stretching of the cervical ligaments due to indirect or direct force applied to a joint (direct forces are rare but do occur); overuse.
Symptoms	Pain on active movement; pain on passive stress of the joint; loss of neck range of motion; tenderness.
Signs	Point tenderness over the cervical spine; swelling; loss of function possible in cases that have associated ligament instability; possible deformity with third-degree injury; possible instability with second- and third-degree injury; inflammation.
Special Tests	Active and resistive movements; passive stress.
Referral/ Diagnostic Procedure	Refer to a physician for clearance for athlete to play if symptoms/signs persist.
Classification of Injury	First-, second-, and third-degree. See Chapter 1 for classification of sprain injuries.

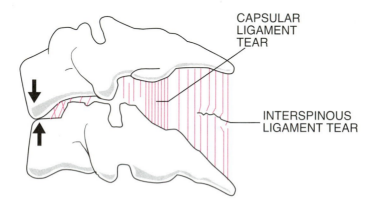

Sprain of ligaments due to hyperflexion of cervical vertebrae.

Medical Term	**Cervical strain**
Common Term	Strained neck
Mechanisms	Indirect trauma to the musculotendinous unit due to excessive forcible contraction or stretching, such as sudden unexpected tackle to athlete.
Symptoms	Pain increased with active movement; pain on passive stretch; loss of function; tenderness. A snapping sound may have been heard when the injury occurred.
Signs	Muscle spasm; swelling; point tenderness; loss of function; loss of strength; hematoma formation; inflammation; head tilted toward the side of the injury.
Special Tests	Active and resistive movements; passive stretch.
Referral/ Diagnostic Procedure	Refer to a physician if symptoms/signs persist.
Classification of Injury	First-, second-, and third-degree. See Chapter 1 for classification of strain injuries.

Medical Term	**Acute torticollis**
Common Term	Wryneck/stiff neck
Mechanisms	In athletics, indirect trauma to the head or neck resulting in local strain with acute spasm. Other possible mechanisms are poor sleeping habits; holding the neck in an unusual position for an extended period of time.
Symptoms	Pain and loss of function due to muscle spasm; tenderness.
Signs	Loss of range of motion due to muscle spasm; restriction of movement to the side opposite of the injury; muscle spasm; head tilted toward the side of the injury; tenderness.
Special Tests	Active and resistive movements; passive stretch.
Referral/ Diagnostic Procedure	Refer to a physician if symptoms/signs persist.
Classification of Injury	Not applicable

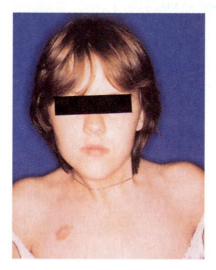

Acute torticollis causing the head to lean to the side of the injury due to muscle spasm.

■ TESTS FOR THE EVALUATION OF THE NECK ■

■ TESTS TO INCREASE INTRATHECAL PRESSURE

Valsalva Test

The athlete is in the sitting position and is asked to bear down as if trying to have a bowel movement. If this causes pain, there is intrathecal pressure or injury involving the theca.

■ CERVICAL SPINE SPECIAL TEST

Distraction Test

The athletic trainer places one hand under the athlete's chin, and the other palm at the base of the skull. Then the athletic trainer gradually lifts (distracts) the head to remove its weight from the neck. Distraction should help relieve the pain in the cervical spine.

Compression Test

The athletic trainer presses down on the top of the athlete's head. If there is an increase in the pain, the athlete should be referred to a physician.

■ NEUROLOGIC ASSESSMENT (Neurologic tests will test muscles, reflexes, and sensory areas.)

Nerve	**C5**
Muscle	Deltoid, Biceps
Test	*Deltoid:* shoulder flexion, abduction, extension
	Biceps: elbow flexion
Reflex	Biceps
Sensory	Lateral arm
Nerve	**C6**
Muscle	Wrist extensor group
Test	Wrist extension
Reflex	Brachioradialis
Sensory	Lateral forearm

95

Nerve	C7
Muscle	Triceps, wrist flexors
Test	*Triceps* Elbow extension
	Wrist flexors Wrist flexion
Reflex	Triceps
Sensory	Middle finger

Nerve	C8
Muscle	Finger flexors
Test	Finger flexion
Reflex	None
Sensory	Ring finger and little finger of the hand and to the distal half of the forearm and the ulna side.

Nerve	T1
Muscle	Finger abductors
Test	Finger abduction
Reflex	None
Sensory	Middle arm

Refer to the Elbow chapter for testing of the radial, ulna, and median nerves.

Range of motion movements

Flexion, extension, rotation, lateral bending. *Note:* If the athlete cannot perform active range of motion tests, passive range of motion tests should not be performed and the athlete should be referred for further assessment by a physician.

■ SPECIAL ASSESSMENT FOR JOINT RANGE OF ■ MOTION AND STRENGTH FOR STRAIN, TENDINITIS, AND TENOSYNOVITIS

Active Movement

The athlete moves the body part through the range of motion actively, trying to reproduce the pain.

Resistive Movement

The athlete moves the body part through the range of motion while the athletic trainer applies resistance.

■ SPECIAL ASSESSMENT FOR JOINT RANGE OF ■ MOTION AND LIGAMENTOUS STABILITY FOR A SPRAIN

Active Movement

The athlete moves the joint through the range of motion actively. The athletic trainer should be looking for any limitations in the range of motion.

Resistive Movement

The athlete moves the joint through the range of motion while the athletic trainer applies resistance.

■ BRACHIAL PLEXUS EVALUATION ■

Evaluation Guide to Neurologic Levels in the Upper Extremity

SPINAL NERVE	C5	C6	C7	C8	T1
Motor	Shoulder adduction, elbow flexion	Wrist extension	Elbow extension, wrist flexion, finger extension	Finger flexion	Finger abduction and adduction
Sensory	Lateral arm	Lateral forearm, thumb, index finger	Middle finger	Medial forearm, ring and small finger	Medial arm
Reflexes	Biceps	Brachio-radialis	Triceps		

Differentiation between Brachial Plexus and Nerve Root Lesions

BRACHIAL PLEXUS LESIONS	NERVE ROOT LESIONS
1. Numbness and burning of entire arm, hand, and fingers.	1. Numbness and burning confined to one or more definable dermatomes.
2. Sensation loss over two to four dermatomes.	2. Sensation loss confined to a definable dermatome.
3. Complete transient paralysis of the arm.	3. Partial transient paralysis of the arm.
4. Tenderness over brachial plexus.	4. No tenderness over brachial plexus.
5. No tenderness over neck posteriorly.	5. Tenderness over neck posteriorly.
6. Increase in symptoms with passive movement of head and neck to *opposite side*.	6. Hyperflexion, extension, or lateral flexion of neck to *same side* as the symptoms may reproduce the symptoms.
7. Symptoms do not occur with downward pressure on head with chin in the supraclavicular fossa.	7. Symptoms occur with downward pressure on head with chin in supraclavicular fossa on same side as lesion.

■ PATHOLOGIC REFLEX TEST ■

Babinski Test

Run a sharp object across the plantar aspect of the foot from the calcaneus along the lateral border to the forefoot. If the great toe extends while the other toes plantar flex, the test is positive.

Oppenheim Test

Run a sharp object along the crest of the tibia. Normally there should be no reaction, but a positive test has the same reaction as the Babinski test.

SHOULDER INJURIES AND CONDITIONS

Chapter 5

Subacromion Bursitis
Subdeltoid Bursitis
Clavicle Contusion
Deltoid Contusion
Long Thoracic Nerve Contusion
Clavicle Fracture
Scapula Fracture
Glenoid Labrum Tear
Rotator Cuff Impingement
Subcoracoid Glenohumeral Luxation
Glenohumeral/Subglenoid Luxation

Long Head of the Biceps Luxation
Posterior Glenohumeral Luxation
Anterior Glenohumeral Subluxation
Posterior Glenohumeral Subluxation
Long Head of the Biceps Rupture
Acromioclavicular Sprain
Strernoclavicular Sprain
Glenohumeral Sprain
Rotator Cuff Strain
Tenosynovitis of the Shoulder

Medical Term	**Subacromion bursitis**
Common Term	Bursitis
Mechanisms	Direct trauma; overuse; stress in throwing; a fall on an outstretched hand.
Symptoms	Pain; loss of function; aching pain at rest; tenderness; night pain.
Signs	Redness; swelling; loss of function; inflammation; pain on rotation; tenderness; pain on abduction greater than 80°; tenderness anterior to acromion and lateral under deltoid at greater tuberosity of the humerus; possible calcium deposits in chronic cases.
Special Tests	Apley's scratch test; resistive movements test.
Referral/ Diagnostic Procedure	Refer to a physician if symptoms/signs persist.
Classification of Injury	First-, second-, or third-degree. See Chapter 1 for classification of bursitis.

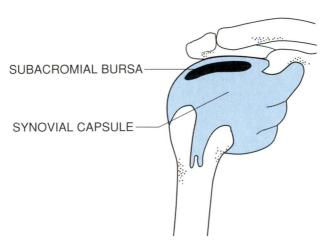

SUBACROMIAL BURSA

SYNOVIAL CAPSULE

Location of subacromial bursa.

Medical Term	**Subdeltoid bursitis**
Common Term	Bursitis
Mechanisms	Direct trauma, such as a fall on an outstretched hand; overuse.
Symptoms	Pain; loss of function; tenderness.
Signs	Redness; swelling; loss of function; tenderness under the deltoid; inflammation; pain and/or weakness on abduction; possible calcium deposits in chronic cases.
Special Tests	Apley's scratch test; resistive movements tests.
Referral/ Diagnostic Procedure	Refer to a physician if symptoms/signs persist.
Classification of Injury	First-, second-, and third-degree. See Chapter 1 for classification of bursitis.

Medical Term	**Clavicle contusion**
Common Term	Bruised collar bone
Mechanisms	Direct trauma to the clavicle.
Symptoms	Pain; loss of function; transitory paralysis; point tenderness.
Signs	Point tenderness; ecchymosis with second- and third-degree injury; hematoma formation; inflammation; loss of function.
Special Tests	Distraction test for acromioclavicular joint stability to rule acromioclavicular sprain.
Referral/ Diagnostic Procedure	Refer to an orthopedic surgeon if symptoms/signs persist. X–ray.
Classification of Injury	First-, second-, and third-degree. See Chapter 1 for classification of contusion.

Medical Term	**Deltoid contusion**
Common Term	Bruised shoulder
Mechanisms	Direct trauma to the deltoid muscle.
Symptoms	Pain; loss of function; transitory paralysis; point tenderness.
Signs	Point tenderness; ecchymosis in second- and third-degree injury; hematoma formation; inflammation; loss of function; weakness on shoulder abduction.
Special Tests	Apley's scratch test; active and resistive abduction.
Referral/ Diagnostic Procedure	Refer to an orthopedic surgeon if symptoms/signs persist. X–ray.
Classification of Injury	First-, second-, and third-degree. See Chapter 1 for contusion classification.

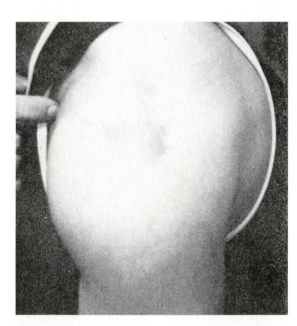

Shoulder contusion (shoulder pointer) with discoloration at the tip of the shoulder due to direct contact.

Medical Term	**Long thoracic nerve contusion**
Common Term	Winging scapula
Mechanisms	Damage to the long thoracic nerve at root level or along the course of the nerve due to indirect trauma to the shoulder or lateral thoracic wall; overuse of the shoulder; prolonged traction, as in cycling.
Symptoms	Dull ache around the shoulder girdle; decrease active in shoulder motion.
Signs	Protruding scapula posteriorly.
Special Tests	Scapula protraction test (pushing against a wall) should cause winging effect.
Referral/ Diagnostic Procedure	Refer of a physician for evaluation. Electromyography (EMG) study.
Classification of Injury	Not applicable

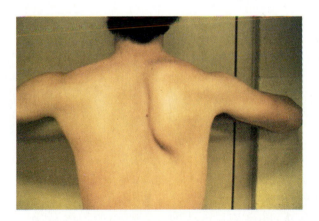

Winging of the scapula due to weakness of the serratus anterior muscle after injury to the long thoracic nerve.

Medical Term	**Clavicle fracture**
Common Term	Broken collar bone
Mechanisms	Fall on an outstretched arm or the tip of the shoulder; direct contact.
Symptoms	Sudden pain; loss of shoulder function; direct and indirect tenderness.
Signs	Loss of shoulder function; rapid swelling; direct and indirect tenderness; possible bony deviations; possible crepitus; possible false joint motion; delayed ecchymosis; head tilted toward the side of the fracture; rounded shoulder. The athlete may be supporting the affected elbow with the opposite hand.
Special Tests	Not applicable
Referral/ Diagnostic Procedure	Refer to an orthopedic surgeon. X–ray.
Classification of Injury	Not applicable

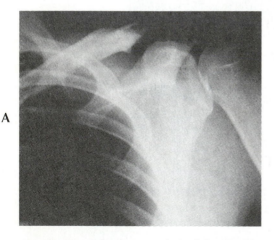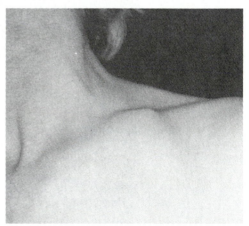

A, AP view of a fractured clavicle. B, Observation of a fractured clavicle normally reveals this appearance of bony deformity.

Medical Term	**Scapula fracture**
Common Term	Cracked or broken shoulder blade
Mechanisms	Direct trauma; indirect trauma from a fall on the arm or shoulder.
Symptoms	Sudden pain; loss of shoulder function; direct and indirect tenderness.
Signs	Loss of shoulder function; rapid swelling; direct and indirect tenderness; possible bony deviations; possible crepitus; possible false joint motion; delayed ecchymosis.
Special Tests	Not applicable
Referral/ Diagnostic Procedure	Refer to an orthopedic surgeon. X–ray.
Classification of Injury	Not applicable

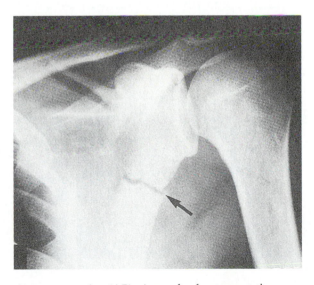

Anteroposterior (AP) view of a fracture at the
lateral border of the scapula *(arrow)*.

Medical Term	**Glenoid labrum tear**
Common Term	Same as above
Mechanisms	Repetition of shoulder motion; acute trauma; anterior subluxation of the glenohumeral joint; anterior instability during acceleration or deceleration phase of throwing due to the biceps tendon pulling on the anterior labrum.
Symptoms	Pain changes the smooth motion of the shoulder; the athlete feels or hears a pop or snap on forced external rotation; the athlete has pain on external rotation at 90° of abduction.
Signs	Loss of smooth shoulder motion; possible positive clunk test; pain on external rotation at 90° of abduction; pain on forced abduction; pain on forced horizontal adduction of the shoulder; weakness of the rotator cuff.
Special Tests	Clunk test; resistive range of motion test, apprehension test.
Referral/ Diagnostic Procedure	Refer to an orthopedic surgeon. MRI and arthrogram.
Classification of Injury	Not applicable

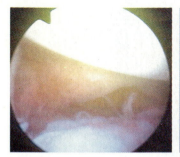 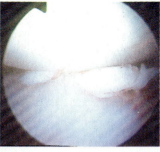 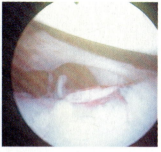

A   B   C

A, Arthoscopic view of a tear in the anterior labrum and capsule after an anterior luxation of the glenohumeral joint. **B**, Arthroscopic view of a torn and avulsed anterior labrum after an anterior luxation of the glenohumeral join. **C**, Arthroscopic view of a central labrial tear and defect after an anterior luxation of the glenohumeral joint.

Medical Term	Rotator cuff impingement
Common Term	Swimmer's shoulder, thrower's shoulder; also occurs in baseball and gymnastics.
Mechanisms	Chronic microtrauma; vascular impairment; partial tear in the rotator cuff muscles.
Symptoms	Increase in pain from internal to external rotation; pain on superolateral aspect of the shoulder; snapping sensation that may be felt with use; loss of function.
Signs	Pain on active abduction between 70° and 130°; pain on extreme forward flexion with the forearm supinated; pain on internal rotation with the arm abducted at 90° and the forearm pronated.
Special Tests	Impingement test; forward flexion test, empty can test, resistive range of motion test.
Referral/ Diagnostic Procedure	Refer to an orthopedic surgeon if symptoms/signs persist.
Classification of Injury	First-, second-, and third-degree. See Chapter 1 for classification of injury.

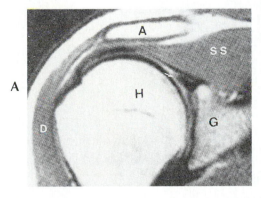
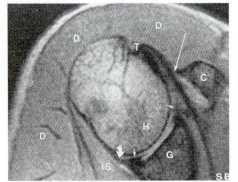

A, Anatomic coronal plane MRI of right shoulder along longitudinal axis of the supraspinatus muscle/tendon. The supraspinatus, subscapularis, and deltoid muscles are visualized extending within the subacromial space and inserting into the greater tuberosity. **B**, Magnetic resonance axial image of right shoulder. At the base and below the coracoid process, the glenohumeral articulation and the glenoid labrum (short arrows) and the subscapularis, infraspinatus, and deltoid muscles are visualized. *A*, Acromion; *G*, glenoid; *H*, humeral head.

Medical Term	**Subcoracoid glenohumeral luxation**
Common Term	Dislocated shoulder—anterior
Mechanisms	Force applied to an abducted, externally rotated arm that is above 90°.
Symptoms	Pain; loss of shoulder function.
Signs	Marked deformity; loss of shoulder function; swelling; point tenderness on the anterior aspect of the shoulder; flattened deltoid; arm fixed in slight abduction and externally rotated.
Special Tests	Check for pulse at the wrist; check sensation over axillary nerve for possible involvement with sensation brush at middle deltoid.
Referral/ Diagnostic Procedure	Refer to an orthopedic surgeon. X–ray.
Classification of Injury	Not applicable

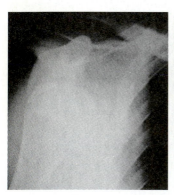 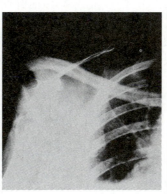 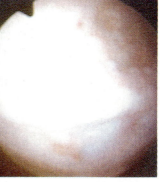

| A | B | C |

A, Subcoracoid (anterior) luxation of the glenohumeral joint indicated by a flattened deltoid and a prominent acromion. **B**, AP view of a subcoracoid luxation; notice the humeral head positioned under the coracoid process. **C**, Arthroscopic view of the head of the humerus, indicating a Hill-Sacks lesion on the head of the humerus after an anterior luxation of the glenohumeral joint.

Medical Term	Glenohumeral/subglenoid luxation
Common Term	Dislocated shoulder—downward
Mechanisms	Force applied to an abducted arm.
Symptoms	Pain; loss of shoulder function.
Signs	Marked deformity; loss of shoulder function; swelling; point tenderness; flattened deltoid; fullness in the axilla due to humeral head; arm fixed in 45° of abduction.
Special Tests	Check the pulse at the wrist. Check for sensory loss in the arm and hand.
Referral/ Diagnostic Procedure	Refer to an orthopedic surgeon. X– ray.
Classification of Injury	Not applicable

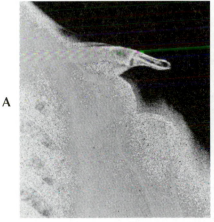 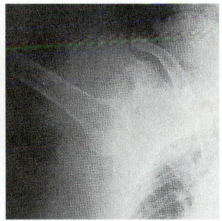

A B

A, X–ray of a subglenoid luxation with the humeral head positioned inferior to the glenoid fossa with the arm fixed in abduction. B, X–ray of a subglenoid luxation of the glenohumeral joint with the humeral head lying inferior to the glenoid fossa.

Medical Term	**Long head of the biceps luxation**
Common Term	Same as above
Mechanisms	Faulty techniques in activity; inadequate muscle development; overuse in throwing; secondary to shallow bicipital groove of the humerus.
Symptoms	Pain in the anterior aspect of the shoulder; loss of shoulder function; snapping sensation followed by a dull ache in the arm or the arm feeling dead.
Signs	Tenderness over the bicipital groove; loss of function; inflammation.
Special Tests	Yergason test, Speed's test, Ludington test, Abbott–Saunders test.
Referral/ Diagnostic Procedure	Refer to a physician.
Classification of Injury	Not applicable

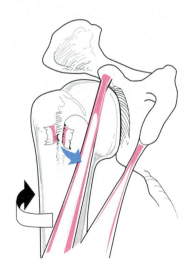

Depiction of dislocation of long head of biceps tendon due to external rotation of the humerus with complete tear of the transverse ligament.

Medical Term	**Posterior glenohumeral luxation**
Common Term	Dislocated shoulder—posterior
Mechanisms	Fall on an outstretched arm; blow to the front of the shoulder.
Symptoms	Pain; loss of shoulder function.
Signs	Marked deformity; loss of shoulder function; swelling; point tenderness; flattened deltoid; arm fixed in adduction and internally rotated. The athletic trainer can palpate the head of the humerus posterior.
Special Tests	Check the pulse at the wrist; check sensation of arm and hand with a sensation brush.
Referral/ Diagnostic Procedure	Refer to an orthopedic surgeon. X–ray.
Classification of Injury	Not applicable

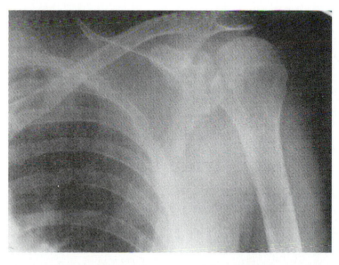

AP view of a posterior luxation of the shoulder, showing the humeral head positioned behind the glenoid fossa.

Medical Term	**Anterior glenohumeral subluxation**
Common Term	Slipping shoulder
Mechanisms	Leverage force applied to an abducted and externally rotated arm.
Symptoms	Pain; loss of function; sensation of the shoulder slipping out of place.
Signs	Obvious deformity before reduction; loss of function; spasm; positive apprehension test. The head of the humerus is palpable slipping forward on the glenoid rim.
Special Tests	Apprehension test; relocation test; sulcus sign; glenohumeral translation test; clunk test.
Referral/ Diagnostic Procedure	Refer to an orthopedic surgeon.
Classification of Injury	Not applicable

Medical Term	**Posterior glenohumeral subluxation**
Common Term	Slipping shoulder
Mechanisms	Posterior force applied to the arm with flexion of the shoulder at 50° to 60°.
Symptoms	Pain; loss of function; clunk sensation on flexion of the shoulder in the posterior aspect; pain decreased by changing arm position.
Signs	The humerus head is prominent posteriorly before reduction. Other signs include slightly flattened deltoid anteriorly, spasm, and loss of function.
Special Tests	Glenohumeral translation test; posterior shoulder instability test; clunk test.
Referral/ Diagnostic Procedure	Refer to an orthopedic surgeon.
Classification of Injury	Not applicable

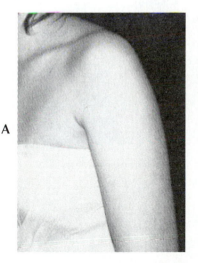 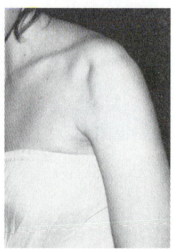

A, Reduced posterior subluxation of the glenohumeral joint. **B**, Posterior subluxation of the glenohumeral joint. Indention is caused by contraction of the anterior deltoid and pectoralis muscles with simultaneous relaxation of the posterior deltoid and external rotators.

Medical Term	**Long head of the biceps rupture**
Common Term	Shoulder strain or biceps tear
Mechanisms	Violent contraction against firm resistance.
Symptoms	Sudden pain; loss of function of the biceps. The athlete hears/feels a sensation of something rolling up the arm.
Signs	Protruding bulge in the biceps, definite loss of strength in the biceps on elbow flexion, tenderness along the long head of the biceps.
Special Tests	Ludington's test.
Referral/ Diagnostic Procedure	Refer to an orthopedic surgeon.
Classification of Injury	Third-degree strain.

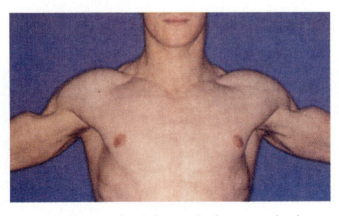

Defective biceps. The defect in the biceps is clearly seen, but is of little functional significance.

Medical Term	**Acromioclavicular sprain**
Common Term	Separated shoulder
Mechanisms	Downward force on the point of the shoulder with the arm adducted; stretching of the acromioclavicular ligament/coracoclavicular ligaments due to direct or indirect force applied to the joint.
Symptoms	Pain on active and resistive movement; pain on passive stress; loss of function; tenderness over the acromioclavicular joint.
Signs	Point tenderness; swelling; hemorrhage; ecchymosis; inflammation; pain on abduction of the shoulder; pain on distraction of the acromioclavicular joint. Abnormal motion of distal clavicle, deformity, and possible instability with second- and third-degree injury.
Special Tests	Distraction test (piano key); cross arm test; pain on abduction; active and resistive movements.
Referral/ Diagnostic Procedure	Refer to an orthopedic surgeon. X–ray.
Classification of Injury	First-, second-, and third-degree. See Chapter 1 for classification of sprain.

See illustrations on p. 120.

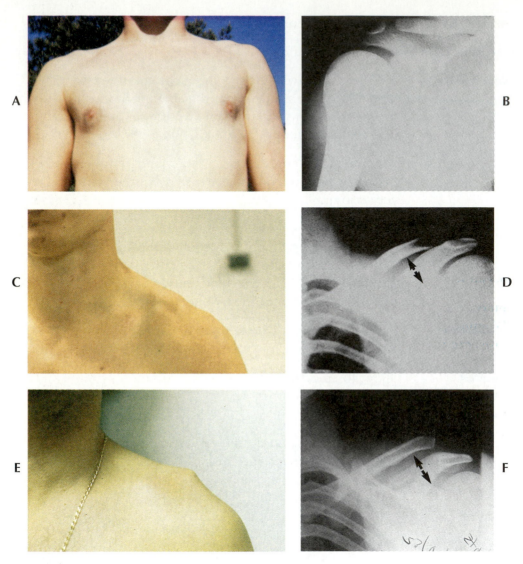

A, First-degree sprain of the right acromioclavicular joint with minimal swelling. The joint has normal appearance. **B**, AP view of the acromioclavicular joint appears normal with a first-degree sprain with a normal joint alignment. **C**, Second-degree sprain of the acromioclavicular joint with moderate swelling and displacement of the clavicle. **D**, AP view of the acromioclavicular joint in a second-degree sprain shows a widening of the AC joint, less than 50%, and a normal spacing of the coracoclavicular joint *(dark arrows)*. **E**, Third-degree sprain of the acromioclavicular joint with a luxation of the distal end of the clavicle. **F**, AP view of the acromioclavicular joint in a third-degree sprain shows a widening of the AC joint, more than 50%, and widening of the coracoclavicular joint *(arrows)*.

Medical Term	**Sternoclavicular sprain**
Common Term	Sprain
Mechanisms	Force applied to the lateral aspect of the shoulder, traveling medially through the clavicle; force applied anterior or posterior to the shoulder; stretching of the sternoclavicular ligament from a direct or indirect force applied to the joint.
Symptoms	Point tenderness over the sternoclavicular joint; pain on active movement and passive stress; loss of function.
Signs	Inflammation; hemorrhage; ecchymosis; deformity possible; instability with second- and third-degree injury.
Special Tests	Active and resistive movements test; passive stress.
Referral/ Diagnostic Procedure	Refer to an orthopedic surgeon. If posterior dislocation, must be concerned with respiratory or vascular impairment. X–ray.
Classification of Injury	First-, second-, and third-degree. See Chapter 1 for classification of sprain.

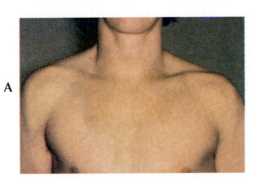
A
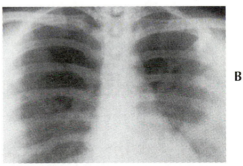
B

A, Sternoclavicular subluxation—clinical appearance. A relatively unusual condition, difficult to treat if the joint becomes clinically unstable. **B**, Note the superior displacement of the clavicle due to the sprain of the sternoclavicular joint.

Medical Term	**Glenohumeral sprain**
Common Term	Sprained shoulder
Mechanisms	Trauma; excessive external rotation force applied to an abducted arm; stretching of the ligament due to direct or indirect force applied to a joint.
Symptoms	Pain on active movement or passive stress; loss of function.
Signs	Point tenderness over the glenohumeral joint; swelling; hemorrhage; possible luxation with third-degree injury; possible instability with second- and third-degree injury; inflammation; ecchymosis.
Special Tests	Sulcus sign; apprehension test; relocation test; glenohumeral translation test; clunk test.
Referral/ Diagnostic Procedure	Refer to a physician if symptoms/signs persist.
Classification of Injury	First-, second-, and third-degree. See Chapter 1 for classification of sprain injury.

Medical Term	**Rotator cuff strain**
Common Term	Same as above
Mechanisms	Trauma to the musculotendinous unit due to excessive forcible contraction or stretching; muscle fatigue may be a predisposing factor; overuse activities.
Symptoms	Pain increased with active movement; pain on passive stretch; loss of function; possible snapping sound when the injury occurs; muscle fatigue before the injury occurs; pain with resistive movements; tenderness.
Signs	Spasm; swelling; ecchymosis; point tenderness over the rotator cuff tendons; loss of strength and function; inflammation; hematoma formation and muscle defect and possible calcium formation with third-degree injury; pain on abduction, external rotation, and flexion of the shoulder.
Special Tests	Apley's scratch test; impingement test; drop arm test; forward flexion test; empty can test.
Referral/ Diagnostic Procedure	Refer to an orthopedic surgeon if symptoms/signs persist.
Classification of Injury	First-, second-, and third-degree. See Chapter 1 for classification of strain injury.

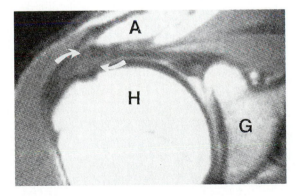

MRI showing swelling from tendinitis in the supraspinatus tendon *(curved arrows)*. A = acromion, H = humeral head, and G = glenoid.

Medical Term	**Tenosynovitis of the shoulder**
Common Term	Same as above
Mechanisms	Overuse; direct trauma; repeated trauma; poor throwing mechanics.
Symptoms	Pain on active and resistive movement; pain on passive stretch; loss of function; tenderness.
Signs	Swelling; thickening of the tendon in chronic cases; snowball crepitus; inflammation; loss of function at rest that increases with activity; tenderness over the tendon.
Special Tests	Active, passive, and resistive range of motion test.
Referral/ Diagnostic Procedure	Refer to an orthopedic surgeon.
Classification of Injury	See Chapter 1 for definition of tenosynovitis.

■ TESTS FOR THE EVALUATION OF INJURIES TO THE SHOULDER ■

■ Tests for Active Range of Motion

Apley's Stretch Test *(Repeat all tests bilaterally.)*

Have the athlete touch the opposite acromion with the hand of the affected shoulder. (Adduction and internal rotation)

Have the athlete put both arms behind the neck and push the elbows backward. (Abduction and external rotation)

Have the athlete raise the arms into abduction, and at 90° supinate the hand and move into full abduction. (Abduction)

Have the athlete touch the inferior border of the opposite scapula. (Abduction and internal rotation)

Have the athlete put both arms behind the back and reach as high as possible. (Abduction and internal rotation)

Have the athlete reach behind the neck and touch the superior border of the opposite scapula. (Adduction and external rotation)

■ Tests for Active and Resistive Movements

(Have the athlete perform these tests actively and against resistance.)

Flexion and Extension Test

With the elbow flexed at 90°, have the athlete actively flex and extend the shoulder. If the athlete can actively do this, repeat the test with manual resistance applied by the athletic trainer. The test should be performed bilaterally.

Abduction and Adduction Test

Have the athlete actively abduct and adduct the arm. If the athlete can do this, repeat the test with manual resistance applied by the athletic trainer. The test should be applied bilaterally.

Internal and External Rotation Test

Have the athlete actively internally and externally rotate the shoulder with the elbow flexed and the shoulder abducted at 90°. If the athlete can do this, repeat the test with manual resistance applied by the athletic trainer. The test should be performed bilaterally.

Scapular Elevation Test

Have the athlete shrug the shoulders against resistance.

Scapular Retraction Test

Place the athletic trainer's hands around the acromion and roll the athlete's shoulders forward; then instruct the athlete to move the shoulders backward, as if standing at attention.

Scapular Protraction Test

Have the athlete stand facing a wall, place palms against the wall in an internally rotated position, and push.

■ Tests for Glenohumeral Stability

Clunk Test

This test is described under *Special Tests for Glenoid Labrum Tears.*

Apprehension Test

Abduct the athlete's shoulder above 90° and externally rotate the arm. If the athlete has anterior instability of the glenohumeral joint, he or she will be very apprehensive about the maneuver. Perform the test bilaterally. Pain will occur anteriorly.

Sulcus Sign

This test is also called a distraction test for the acromioclavicular joint. The athlete sits with both arms hanging by his or her sides. The athletic trainer grasps the wrist and pulls down, then looks for a hollowing out just distal to the joint. The test should be performed bilaterally.

Relocation Test

Abduct the athlete's shoulder above 90° and externally rotate the arm, as in the apprehension test. Then apply an anterior force to the humeral head to test for anterior instability. Perform the test bilaterally.

Posterior Stability Test

With the athlete in the supine position, the athletic trainer grasps the humeral head, holding the athlete's elbow with the opposite hand. The athletic trainer tries to move the humeral head posteriorly to demonstrate posterior instability. The athletic trainer can also try to move the humeral head anteriorly to demonstrate anterior instability. The test should be performed bilaterally.

Glenohumeral Translation Test

The athlete is supine or sitting. The athletic trainer grasps the humeral head while stabilizing the scapula, and moves the humeral head in an anterior and posterior movement to determine anterior and posterior instability of the shoulder. The test should be performed bilaterally.

■ Special Test for Rotator Cuff Injuries

Forward Flexion Test

Have the athlete move the shoulder into extreme forward flexion with the hand in a supinated position. Pain in the anterior shoulder indicates possible impingement of the rotator cuff.

Impingement Test

The athletic trainer abducts, forward flexes, and internally rotates the athlete's shoulder, causing impingement of the supraspinatus tendon on the acromion and coracoacromial ligament, reproducing the athlete's pain. Pain indicates a possible impingement of the rotator cuff.

Empty Can Test

Have the athlete abduct the arm at 90°, internally rotate the arm, and move to 30° of horizontal adduction. The athletic trainer pushes down on the athlete's arms while the athlete resists the pressure. Pain indicates a possible impingement or injury to the supraspinatus muscle.

Drop Arm Test

With the athlete standing, have him or her abduct the arms as high as possible against gravity, then lower the arms to approximately 90° of abduction. If the supraspinatus tendon is torn, the arm will drop to the side. The athletic trainer can apply a tap to the wrist to reproduce the pain.

■ Special Test for Acromioclavicular Joint

Distraction Test (Piano Key Sign)

The athlete sits with both arms hanging by his or her side. The athletic trainer grasps the wrist and pulls down, then looks for a hollowing-out just distal to the joint. The test should be performed bilaterally.

Crossover Maneuver

The athletic trainer passively abducts the athletes arm across the front of the athlete's body, compressing the joint.

■ Special Test for Glenoid Labrum Tears

Clunk Test

With the athlete in the supine position, the athletic trainer stands superior to the shoulder and moves the arm from 90° of abduction to full abduction, beginning with the arm externally rotated at 90°. The athletic trainer places one hand at the elbow, applying pressure against the humerus, while the other hand is placed over the glenohumeral joint, with the thumb on the anterior surface of the joint, feeling for a "clunk" or popping sensation. The humerus is internally and externally rotated as the arm is moved into full abduction. This test can also be used for testing stability of the glenohumeral joint. The test should be performed bilaterally.

■ Test for Biceps Tendon Stability

Yergason Test

The athlete can be sitting or standing; the elbow is flexed at 90° and the forearm is pronated. The athletic trainer places one hand on the elbow and the other hand at the athlete's wrist. The athlete is instructed to hold this position while the athletic trainer tries to externally rotate and extend the elbow.

Abbott-Saunders Test

The athlete is in the sitting position; the athletic trainer fully abducts and externally rotates the athlete's arm. The athletic trainer then lowers the athlete's arm to the side. A palpable or audible click indicates a subluxation or dislocation of the biceps tendon.

■ Test of Biceps Tendinitis

Speed's Test

Athletic trainer resist flexion of the shoulder by the athlete. The athlete's forearm is supinated and the elbow is completed extended. A positive test indicates tenderness in the bicipital groove.

■ Test for Biceps Tendon Rupture

Ludington's Test

Have the athlete sit and place both hands behind the head, grasping the fingers together, then contract and relax the biceps. The athletic trainer feels for deviation in the biceps.

■ Test for Thoracic Outlet Syndrome

Adson Test

This test is used to determine the state of the subclavian artery. The athletic trainer takes the athlete's radial pulse at the wrist, then adducts, extends, and externally rotates the arm. He or she then instructs the athlete to take a deep breath and turn the head toward the arm being tested. The trainer should feel for a reduction or absence of the pulse. If the pulse is reduced, this indicates a compression of the artery by an extra cervical rib or tightened scalenus muscle. This test is also referred to as the anterior scalene syndrome test.

Costoclavicular Syndrome Test

This test indicates whether the subclavian artery is being compressed between the first rib and the clavicle. The athlete stands at attention, the shoulders are in posterior abduction, the arm is extended, and the neck is hyperextended. If the pulse is reduced or absent, the test is positive.

Hyperabduction Syndrome Test

The athletic trainer takes the athlete's radial pulse, while the athlete raises both hands and fully extends the arms over the head. This tests the subclavian artery and axillary vessels and the brachial plexus. If there is a reduction or absence of the radial pulse, the test is positive.

■ Test for Winging of the Scapula

Scapula Protraction Test

The athlete stands with feet approximately one foot from a wall. With the arm abducted at 90°, the elbows flexed, the athlete leans toward the wall, placing the hands against it. He or she then pushes against the wall. If the scapula protrudes outward, the test is positive.

UPPER ARM INJURIES AND CONDITIONS

Chapter 6

Medical Term	**Contusion of biceps**
Common Term	Bruise
Mechanisms	Direct trauma.
Symptoms	Pain; loss of elbow flexion and extension; transitory paralysis of the biceps; point tenderness.
Signs	Ecchymosis; hematoma formation; inflammation; loss of elbow flexion and extension.
Special Tests	Active, passive, resistive range of motion tests.
Referral/ Diagnostic Procedure	Refer of a physician if symptoms/signs persist.
Classification of Injury	First-, second-, and third-degree. See Chapter 1 for classification of contusion injury.

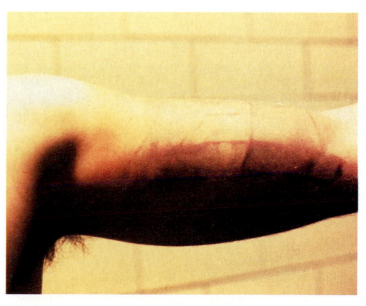

Biceps contusion indicated by swelling and ecchymosis after direct trauma to the biceps.

Medical Term	**Proximal humerus epiphyseal plate injury**
Common Term	Fractured humerus
Mechanisms	Direct trauma; indirect trauma traveling along the length of the humerus.
Symptoms	Sudden pain; loss of function; direct or indirect tenderness.
Signs	Loss of function; possible deformity; rapid swelling; direct tenderness; indirect tenderness; possible bony deviations; possible crepitus; possible false joint; delayed ecchymosis.
Special Tests	Not applicable
Referral/ Diagnostic Procedure	Refer to an orthopedic surgeon. X–ray.
Classification of Injury	See Chapter 1 for classification of epiphyseal plate fracture.

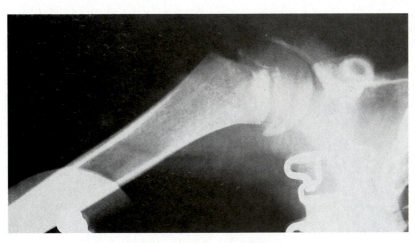

Fracture of proximal humerus epiphyseal plate.

Medical Term	**Exostosis/Myositis ossificans**
Common Term	Blocker's exostosis; tackler's exostosis; blocker's spur
Mechanisms	Repeated trauma to the humerus.
Symptoms	Pain; point tenderness; possible paresthesia.
Signs	Painful bony prominence; swelling; loss of function of elbow flexion and extension.
Special Tests	Not applicable
Referral/ Diagnostic Procedure	Refer to an orthopedic surgeon. X–ray.
Classification of Injury	Not applicable

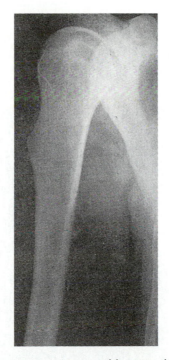

Benign exostosis–a red herring that presented in a patient with overlying referred pain from the cervical spine.

Medical Term	**Humerus fracture**
Common Term	Broken arm
Mechanisms	Direct trauma applied to the arm from a fall or external force; indirect trauma from a fall on an outstretched hand.
Symptoms	Sudden pain; loss of function; direct or indirect tenderness.
Signs	Loss of function; possible deformity; rapid swelling; direct and indirect tenderness; possible bony deviations; possible crepitus; possible false joint motion; delayed ecchymosis; possible shortened humerus.
Special Tests	Not applicable
Referral/ Diagnostic Procedure	Refer to a orthopedic surgeon. X– ray.
Classification of Injury	Not applicable

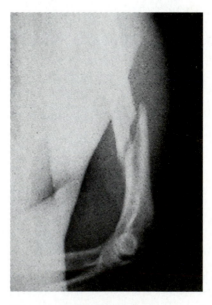

Fracture of the humerus.

Medical Term	Axillary nerve injury
Common Term	Contusion to peripheral nerve
Mechanisms	Direct trauma to the lateral arm, possibly secondary to an anteriorly dislocated shoulder.
Symptoms	Dermatome numbness in area of the middle deltoid; loss of abduction of the shoulder; tenderness.
Signs	Point tenderness; loss of function of the deltoid and biceps.
Special Tests	Sensation brush for change in sensation in middle deltoid; active and resistive range of motion for strength of the deltoid.
Referral/ Diagnostic Procedure	Refer to a neurologist.
Classification of Injury	Not applicable

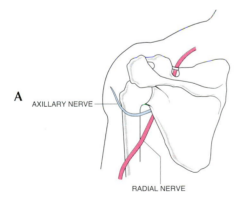
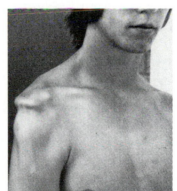

A, Course of the axillary nerve as it travels posterior to the proximal humerus. **B**, Wasting of the deltoid from isolated axillary nerve injury.

Medical Term	**Triceps strain**
Common Term	Pulled arm muscle
Mechanisms	Trauma to the musculotendinous unit due to excessive forcible contraction or stretching; muscle fatigue could be a predisposing mechanism.
Symptoms	Pain with active and resistive elbow extension; pain on passive elbow flexion; possible snapping sensation when the injury occurred; muscle fatigue before the injury occurred; tenderness.
Signs	Spasm; swelling; ecchymosis; point tenderness; inflammation; loss of function and strength. Hematoma formation, possible defect, and possible calcium formation with third-degree injury.
Special Tests	Active and resistive movements; passive stretch.
Referral/ Diagnostic Procedure	Refer to a physician if symptoms/signs persist.
Classification of Injury	First-, second-, and third-degree. See Chapter 1 for classification of strain injury.

Medical Term	Biceps tendinitis
Common Term	Same as above
Mechanisms	Irritation of the biceps tendon in the bicipital groove; repeated microtrauma to the tendon itself or to the muscle–tendon attachments; degenerative changes; overuse activity.
Symptoms	Pain on active and resistive movements; loss of function; overuse activity; pain on passive stretch; tenderness.
Signs	Erythema; swelling; loss of function; inflammation; possible crepitus over the bicipital groove; pain on abduction and external rotation; tenderness; possible calcium formation.
Special Tests	Active and resistive movement; passive stretch; rotator cuff muscle test, since biceps tendon lies close to the subscapularis tendon.
Referral/ Diagnostic Procedure	Refer to a physician if symptoms/signs persist.
Classification of Injury	See Chapter 1 for definition of tendinitis.

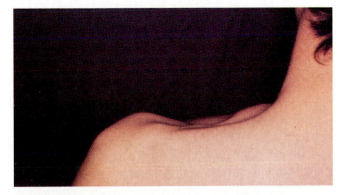

A clinical photograph showing localized swelling over the anterior aspect of the shoulder due to inflammation and effusion into the biceps tendon sheath.

ELBOW INJURIES AND CONDITIONS

Chapter 7

Olecranon Bursitis

Contusion

Lateral Epicondylitis/Radiohumeral
  Bursitis

Medial Epicondylitis

Distal Humerus Epiphyseal Plate
  Injury

Proximal Radius Epiphyseal Plate
  Injury

Proximal Ulna Epiphyseal Plate
  Injury

Distal Humerus Fracture

Radius Fracture

Supercondylar Fracture

Ulna Fracture

Anterior Elbow Luxation

Posterior Elbow Luxation

Ulnar Nerve Contusion

Median Nerve Injury

Radial Nerve Injury

Ulnar Nerve Injury

Osteochondritis Dissecans

Collateral Ligaments Sprain

Volkmann's Contracture

Medical Term	**Olecranon bursitis**
Common Term	Bursitis
Mechanisms	Acute or chronic injury; direct trauma from a fall on a hard surface, such as an artificial surface.
Symptoms	Pain; loss of function; tenderness.
Signs	Redness; swelling; loss of function; point tenderness over the olecranon; inflammation; localized swelling at the olecranon; possible calcium formation in chronic cases.
Special Tests	Not applicable.
Referral/ Diagnostic Procedure	Refer to a physician.
Classification of Injury	See Chapter 1 for description of bursitis.

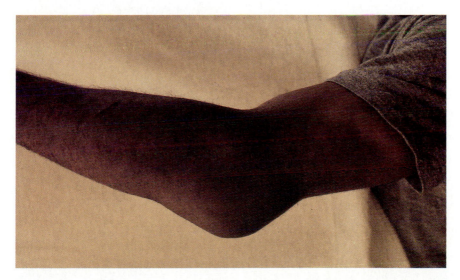

Olecranon bursitis in a football player as a result of falling on an artificial surface.

Medical Term	Contusion
Common Term	Bruised elbow
Mechanisms	Direct trauma.
Symptoms	Pain; loss of elbow function; transitory paralysis; tenderness.
Signs	Point tenderness; ecchymosis; hematoma formation; inflammation; loss of elbow function; possible calcium formation with third-degree contusion.
Special Tests	Active, passive, resistive range of motion test.
Referral/ Diagnostic Procedure	Refer to a physician if symptoms/signs persist.
Classification of Injury	First-, second-, and third-degree. See Chapter 1 for classification of contusion injury.

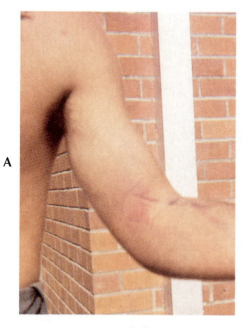 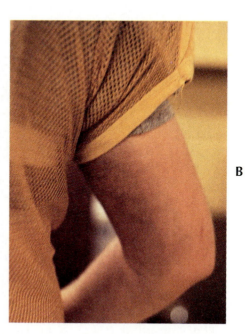

A, Anterior view of elbow contusion. **B**, Swelling and ecchymosis due to direct trauma to the elbow.

Medical Term	Lateral epicondylitis/radiohumeral bursitis
Common Term	Tennis elbow/pitcher's elbow
Mechanisms	Continuous forceful extension of the forearm with pronation as in hitting a backhand stroke in tennis or striking a golf ball with a golf club.
Symptoms	Pain of the lateral epicondyle with wrist extension against resistance; loss of function; tenderness; pain on active and resistive extension of the wrist.
Signs	Point tenderness of the lateral epicondyle; inflammation; loss of function; swelling; pain with extension of the wrist against resistance.
Special Tests	Active and resistive wrist extension test and hand-shaking test.
Referral/ Diagnostic Procedure	Refer to an orthopedist if symptoms/signs persist.
Classification of Injury	See Chapter 1 for classification of sprains.

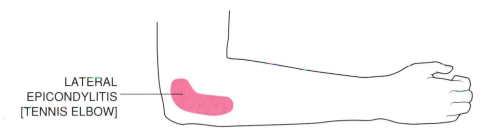

LATERAL
EPICONDYLITIS
[TENNIS ELBOW]

Lateral view of right arm with denoted area of pain of lateral epicondylitis.

Medical Term	**Medial epicondylitis**
Common Term	Tennis elbow/golfer's elbow/Little League elbow
Mechanisms	Overuse; sudden, vigorous supinating movements of the forearm and wrist, as in throwing a curve ball in baseball or serving in tennis.
Symptoms	Pain over the medial epicondyle with forearm pronation and flexion that occurs with both active and resistive movements; symptoms also include loss of function and tenderness; persistent discomfort and stiffness.
Signs	Loss of function; inflammation; swelling; muscle weakness; pain on supination of the forearm and extension of the wrist against resistance; point tenderness over the medial epicondyle.
Special Tests	Medial epicondylitis test.
Referral/ Diagnostic Procedure	Refer to an orthopedist if symptoms/signs persist.
Classification of Injury	See Chapter 1 for classification of sprains.

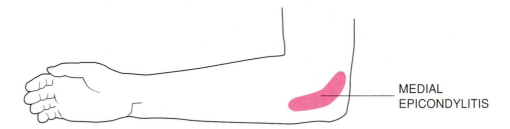

MEDIAL
EPICONDYLITIS

Medial view of right arm with denoted area for medial epicondylitis.

Medical Term	**Distal humerus epiphyseal plate injury**
Common Term	Fracture
Mechanisms	Direct or indirect trauma; a fall on an outstretched hand or hyperextended wrist; repetitious or overuse activities in young athletes.
Symptoms	Sudden pain; loss of function; direct or indirect tenderness.
Signs	Loss of function; possible deformity; rapid swelling; direct or indirect tenderness; possible bony deviation; possible crepitus; possible false joint motion; delayed ecchymosis.
Special Tests	Check radial pulse.
Referral/ Diagnostic Procedure	Refer to an orthopedist. X–ray.
Classification of Injury	See Chapter 1 for classification of epiphyseal plate fractures.

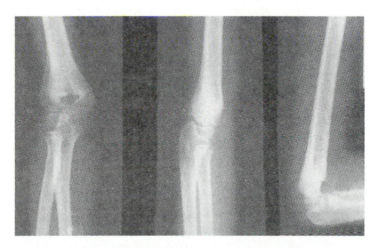

Displaced lower humeral epiphysis (supracondylar fracture) following a fall from gymnastic apparatus.

Medical Term	**Proximal radius epiphyseal plate injury**
Common Term	Fracture
Mechanisms	Direct or indirect trauma; a fall on an outstretched hand or hyperextended wrist.
Symptoms	Sudden pain; loss of function; direct or indirect tenderness.
Signs	Loss of function; possible deformity; rapid swelling; direct or indirect tenderness; possible bony deviation; possible crepitus; possible false joint motion; delayed ecchymosis.
Special Tests	Check radial pulse.
Referral/ Diagnostic Procedure	Refer to an orthopedist. X–ray.
Classification of Injury	See Chapter 1 for classification of epiphyseal plate fracture.

Medical Term	**Proximal ulna epiphyseal plate injury**
Common Term	Fracture
Mechanisms	Direct or indirect trauma; a fall on an outstretched hand or hyperextended wrist.
Symptoms	Sudden pain; loss of function; direct or indirect tenderness.
Signs	Loss of function; possible deformity; rapid swelling; direct or indirect tenderness; possible bony deviations; possible crepitus; possible false joint motion; delayed ecchymosis.
Special Tests	Not applicable
Referral/ Diagnostic Procedure	Refer to an orthopedist. X–ray.
Classification of Injury	See Chapter 1 for classification of epiphyseal plate fracture.

Medical Term	**Distal humerus fracture**
Common Term	Broken arm
Mechanisms	Direct trauma, such as direct contact to the humerus; indirect trauma, such as a fall on an outstretched hand or elbow.
Symptoms	Sudden pain; loss of function; direct or indirect tenderness.
Signs	Loss of function; possible deformity; rapid swelling; direct or indirect tenderness; possible bony deviation; possible crepitus; possible false joint motion; delayed ecchymosis.
Special Tests	Check radial pulse.
Referral/ Diagnostic Procedure	Refer to an orthopedist. X–ray.
Classification of Injury	Not applicable

Medical Term	Radius fracture
Common Term	Broken forearm
Mechanisms	Direct trauma; twisting force, such as in wrestling and gymnastics; or impact force, such as falling on an outstretched hand.
Symptoms	Sudden pain; loss of function; direct or indirect tenderness; numbness or coldness in lower arm if circulation is impaired.
Signs	Loss of function; possible deformity; rapid swelling; direct or indirect tenderness; possible bony deviation; possible crepitus; possible false joint motion; delayed ecchymosis.
Special Tests	Check radial pulse.
Referral/ Diagnostic Procedure	Refer to an orthopedist. X–ray.
Classification of Injury	Not applicable

A 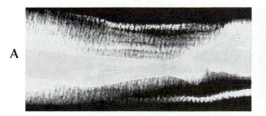 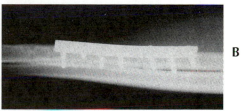 B

A, X-ray of a fractured radius. B, Repair of radius fracture.

Medical Term	**Supercondylar fracture**
Common Term	Fractured elbow
Mechanisms	Indirect trauma from a fall on an outstretched hand and hyperextended elbow; direct trauma from a fall on the elbow.
Symptoms	Sudden pain; loss of function; direct or indirect tenderness.
Signs	Loss of function; possible deformity; rapid swelling; direct or indirect tenderness; possible bony deviation; possible crepitus; possible false joint motion; delayed ecchymosis; possible delayed nerve or vascular injury leading to Volkmann's ischemic contracture.
Special Tests	Check radial pulse.
Referral/ Diagnostic Procedure	Refer to an orthopedist. X–ray.
Classification of Injury	Not applicable

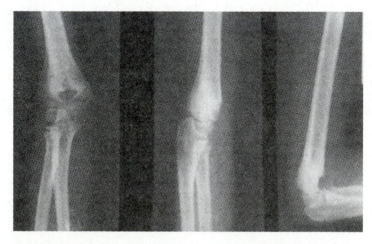

Displaced lower humeral epiphysis (supracondylar fracture) following a fall from gymnastic apparatus.

Medical Term	Ulna fracture
Common Term	Broken forearm
Mechanisms	Direct trauma; indirect or impact force as in a fall on an outstretched hand; twisting force, as in wrestling or gymnastics.
Symptoms	Sudden pain; loss of function; direct or indirect tenderness.
Signs	Loss of function; possible deformity; rapid swelling; direct or indirect tenderness; possible bony deviation; possible crepitus; possible false joint motion; delayed ecchymosis.
Special Tests	Check radial pulse.
Referral/ Diagnostic Procedure	Refer to an orthopedist. X–ray.
Classification of Injury	Not applicable

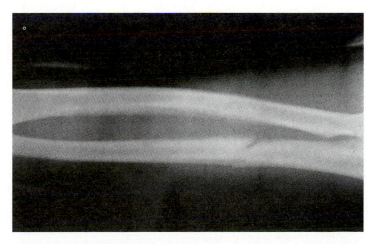

X-ray of a fractured ulna.

Medical Term	**Anterior elbow luxation**
Common Term	Dislocated elbow
Mechanisms	Direct trauma to the elbow.
Symptoms	Pain; loss of function.
Signs	Marked deformity; loss of function; swelling; point tenderness; elbow fixed in extension; absence of olecranon; fullness in the cubital fossa from the condyles of the humerus.
Special Tests	Check the pulse at the wrist, check blood flow at the nail beds, check motor and sensory function of the hand.
Referral/ Diagnostic Procedure	Refer to an orthopedist. X–ray for possible fracture.
Classification of Injury	See Chapter 1 for description of luxation.

Medical Term	**Posterior elbow luxation**
Common Term	Dislocated elbow
Mechanisms	Fall on a hyperextended/flexed elbow with supinated forearm forcing the olecranon process into the olecranon fossa, which forces the trochlea over the coronoid process; severe torsion.
Symptoms	Pain; loss of function.
Signs	Marked deformity; loss of function; swelling; point tenderness; increase in the anterior/posterior diameter of the elbow; the elbow fixed in flexion, prominent olecranon.
Special Tests	Check the pulse at the wrist, check blood flow at the nail beds, check sensory and motor function of the hand.
Referral/ Diagnostic Procedure	Refer to an orthopedist. X–ray for possible fracture.
Classification of Injury	See Chapter 1 for description of luxation.

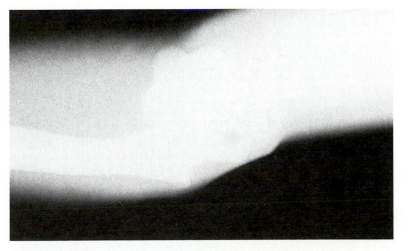

X-ray of a posterior luxation of the elbow, indicated by the prominence of the olecranon.

Medical Term	**Ulnar nerve contusion**
Common Term	Bruised nerve—funny bone
Mechanisms	Direct trauma.
Symptoms	Pain; loss of function; numbness, tingling and/or burning sensation in the forearm and hand over the ulnar nerve distribution.
Signs	Loss of function in the forearm and fourth and fifth fingers.
Special Tests	Sensation and motor test over the ulnar nerve distribution, Tinel's sign.
Referral/ Diagnostic Procedure	Refer to a neurologist if symptoms/signs persist.
Classification of Injury	Not applicable

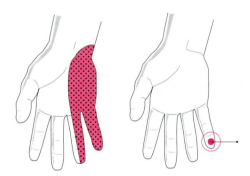

Sign of injury to the ulnar nerve is the loss of sensation in the dotted area with the best area being the tip of the fifth finger.

Medical Term	**Median nerve injury**
Common Term	Contusion to a nerve
Mechanisms	Direct trauma; repetition; compression resulting from a fracture or luxation.
Symptoms	Weakness in grip; muscle atrophy of thenar eminence; numbness.
Signs	Sensory loss in nerve distribution; weakness of thumb abduction against resistance; loss of function.
Special Tests	Thumb abduction against resistance; check sensation on palmar aspect of index finger, tinel's sign.
Referral/ Diagnostic Procedure	Refer to a neurologist if symptoms/signs persist.
Classification of Injury	Not applicable

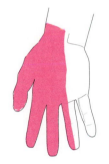 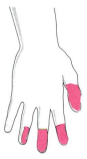

Areas of sensation for the median nerve (shaded area).

Medical Term	**Radial nerve injury**
Common Term	Contusion to a nerve
Mechanisms	Direct trauma; compression of the radial nerve above the elbow from sudden forceful triceps contraction; fractures of the humerus; elbow luxations.
Symptoms	Pain; weakness on finger extension; numbness.
Signs	Sensory loss; muscle weakness on extension of the fingers against resistance.
Special Tests	Test finger extension against resistance; check area of sensation on the dorsum of the hand between the thumb and the index finger, Tinel's sign.
Referral/ Diagnostic Procedure	Refer to a neurologist if symptoms/signs persist.
Classification of Injury	Not applicable

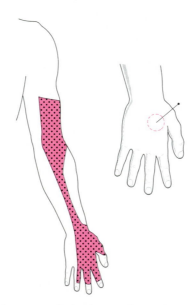

Sign for injury to radial nerve is loss of sensation in dotted area, with the key area being the web space between the thumb and index finger.

Medical Term	**Ulnar nerve injury**
Common Term	Contusion of a nerve
Mechanisms	Direct trauma to the ulnar nerve; entrapment in scar tissue or muscular tissue, repetitive valgus stress to the elbow, as in throwing a baseball; subluxation of the ulnar nerve. Possible cervical spinal nerve root, brachial plexus involvement, or thoracic outlet syndrome.
Symptoms	Muscle weakness; pain on elbow flexion; muscle atrophy; numbness or tingling in the forearm and hand; burning sensation or dead feeling in the forearm or hand.
Signs	Sensory loss over nerve distribution; possible atrophy of muscles; loss of function; impaired abduction and adduction of fifth finger; impaired adduction of thumb and abduction of index finger, Tinel's sign; full elbow flexion for 5 minutes will often reproduce symptoms.
Special Tests	Test abduction and adduction of the fifth finger against resistance; test adduction of thumb and abduction of index finger against resistance; check area of sensation at tip of the fifth finger, Tinel's sign, elbow flexion for 5 minutes.
Referral/ Diagnostic Procedure	Refer to a neurologist if symptoms/signs persist.
Classification of Injury	Not applicable

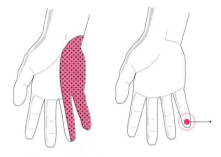

Sign of injury to the ulnar nerve is the loss of sensation in the dotted area with the best area being the tip of the fifth finger.

Medical Term	Osteochondritis dissecans
Common Term	Joint mice
Mechanisms	Unknown; impaired blood supply to area; articular or hyaline cartilage degeneration.
Symptoms	Pain after exercise; loss of function.
Signs	Chronic nonspecific swelling; loss of function; muscle atrophy; possible crepitus; transient locking.
Special Tests	Active, passive, and resistive movements.
Referral/ Diagnostic Procedure	Refer to an orthopedist if symptoms/signs persist. X–ray, MRI.
Classification of Injury	Not applicable

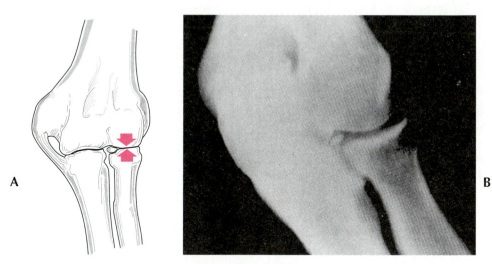

A, Radial head capitellum compression loose bodies. **B**, X-ray of capitellum compression loose bodies.

Medical Term	**Collateral ligaments sprain**
Common Term	Sprain
Mechanisms	Indirect trauma; overuse; forced hyperextension; a valgus force applied to the ulnar collateral ligament or a varus force applied to the radial collateral, stretching the ligament.
Symptoms	Pain on active and resistive movement; passive stress; loss of function; tenderness.
Signs	Point tenderness over a ligament; swelling; hemorrhage; possible deformity with third degree injury; ecchymosis; possible instability with second or third degree injury; inflammation.
Special Tests	Valgus and varus stress test for ligament stability; active and resistive movement.
Referral/ Diagnostic Procedure	Refer to an orthopedist if symptoms/signs persist.
Classification of Injury	First-, second-, and third-degree. See Chapter 1 for classification of sprain.

A 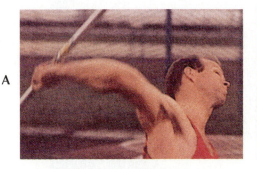 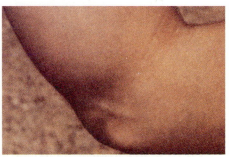 B

A, Mechanism of injury-the "round arm" throw. **B**, Clinical appearance with loss of normal common flexor muscle bulk.

Medical Term	Volkmann's contracture
Common Term	Same as above
Mechanisms	Supracondyle fracture of the humerus.
Symptoms	Pain in the forearm that increases when the fingers are passively extended; paralysis; ischemia and neurologic changes such as coldness, stiffness, or numbness of the fingers.
Signs	Swelling; ecchymosis; possible deformity; possible cessation of brachial and radial pulses; muscle spasm; possible necrosis of forearm muscles due to pressure on brachial artery.
Special Tests	Use of tissue manometers to measure compartment pressure; Allen's test.
Referral/ Diagnostic Procedure	Refer to a orthopedist and neurologist. X–ray.
Classification of Injury	Not applicable

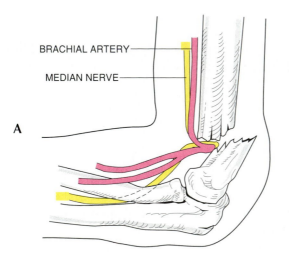
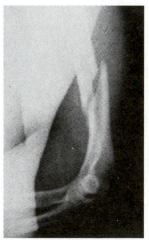

A, Volkmann's contracture is the result of the mechanism of impairment to the vascular supply to the muscles of the forearm.
B, Humerus fracture.

TESTS FOR THE EVALUATION OF INJURIES TO THE ELBOW

TESTS FOR LATERAL EPICONDYLITIS

Wrist Extension Test

The athlete flexes the elbow at 90°, then the athletic trainer applies resistance to the hand as the athlete tries to extend the wrist. A positive test would reproduce the athlete's pain over the lateral epicondyle.

Hand Shaking Test

The athletic trainer tells the athlete to shake hands using the affected arm. A positive test would reproduce the athlete's pain.

TESTS FOR MEDIAL EPICONDYLITIS

Forearm Supination and Wrist and Elbow Extension

The athletic trainer applies resistance to the athlete's affected arm in the movement of supination in the forearm and extension of the wrist and elbow. A positive test would reproduce the athlete's pain.

COLLATERAL LIGAMENTOUS STABILITY TEST

To test the stability of the collateral ligaments of the elbow, the athletic trainer places one hand on the medial side of the elbow joint and the other hand on the lateral side of the distal forearm. He or she then applies a varus force testing the radial collateral ligament, then changes hand position and applies a valgus force testing the ulnar collateral ligament.

SPECIAL TEST FOR ULNAR, MEDIAN, AND RADIAL NERVE DISTRIBUTIONS

Nerve	Ulnar
Sensation	Ulnar side of the hand, both dorsum and palm; lateral side of the fourth finger; all of the fifth finger.
Sensation Test	Tip of the fifth finger, volar surface.
Motor Test	Adduction of the thumb against resistance; abduction of the index finger against resistance; adduction and abduction against resistance of the fourth and fifth fingers.

Test adduction of the fourth and fifth fingers by placing a piece of paper between the fingers and trying to pull it out while the athlete tries to hold on to it.

Nerve	Median
Sensation	Radial portion of the palm and the palm surface of the thumb, index, and middle fingers, and the medial side of the fourth finger; dorsum of the tips of the thumb, index, middle, and fourth fingers.
Sensation Test	Tip of the index finger.
Motor Test	Thumb abduction against resistance.
Nerve	Radial
Sensation	Dorsum of the radial side of the hand; thumb, index finger, middle, and fourth finger to the distal digits.
Sensation Test	Space between the thumb and the index finger.
Motor Test	Extension of the fingers against resistance.

■ SPECIAL TEST FOR VASCULAR OCCLUSION

Allen Test

The athletic trainer instructs the athlete to open and close the hand quickly, several times, then squeeze the fist tightly. The athletic trainer places his or her thumb over the radial artery and the middle finger over the ulnar artery, to occlude the arteries. With the arteries occluded, the athletic trainer tells the athlete to open the hand, then releases one of the arteries. The hand should turn pink as the blood returns to it. This procedure is repeated with the other artery. If the hand does not turn pink, damage to the artery may have occurred.

■ GENERAL ASSESSMENT FOR JOINT RANGE OF MOTION AND STRENGTH FOR STRAIN, TENDINITIS, TENOSYNOVITIS

Active Movement

The athlete moves the body part through the range of motion actively, trying to reproduce the pain.

Passive Stretch

The athletic trainer performs a passive stretch of the involved muscle or tendon.

Resistive Movement

> The athlete moves the body part through the range of motion while the athletic trainer applies resistance.

■ GENERAL ASSESSMENT FOR JOINT RANGE OF MOTION AND STRENGTH FOR STRAIN, TENDINITIS, TENOSYNOVITIS

Active Movement

> The athlete moves the body part through the range of motion actively, trying to reproduce the pain.

Passive Stretch

> The athletic trainer performs a passive stretch of the involved muscle or tendon.

Resistive Movement

> The athlete moves the body part through the range of motion while the athletic trainer applies resistance.

■ GENERAL ASSESSMENT FOR JOINT RANGE OF MOTION AND LIGAMENTOUS STABILITY FOR A SPRAIN

Active Movement

> The athlete moves the joint through the range of motion actively. The athletic trainer should be looking for any limitations in the range of motion.

Passive Movement

> If the athlete cannot move the joint through the range of motion actively, then passive range of motion should be done to determine if the range of motion is blocked due to the athlete's pain or if some object is blocking the joint.

Resistive Movement

> The athlete moves the joint through the range of motion while the athletic trainer applies resistance.

Passive Stress

> The athletic trainer applies stress to the joint to test the integrity of the ligamentous structures of the joint.

WRIST INJURIES AND CONDITIONS

Chapter 8

Medical Term	Navicular (scaphoid) fracture
Common Term	Same as above
Mechanisms	Indirect trauma to an outstretched hand (thumb) or hyperextended wrist.
Symptoms	Sudden pain; loss of function; direct and indirect tenderness.
Signs	Loss of function; rapid swelling; direct tenderness in the anatomic snuffbox; indirect tenderness; possible bony deviation; possible crepitus; possible false motion; delayed ecchymosis.
Special Tests	Compression of thumb; pressure into anatomic snuffbox.
Referral/ Diagnostic Procedure	Refer to an orthopedist. X–ray.
Classification of Injury	Not applicable

A 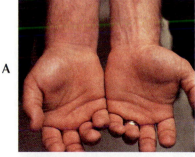 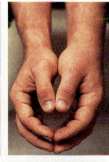 B

C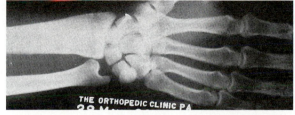

THE ORTHOPEDIC CLINIC PA

A and **B**, Swelling of the wrist in the anatomic snuffbox due to a navicular (scaphoid) fracture. **C**, X-ray showing a repair of a fracture of the navicular.

Medical Term	Colles' fracture
Common Term	Broken wrist
Mechanisms	Indirect trauma or direct trauma to the distal forearm by a fall on an outstretched hand or a hyperextended wrist fracturing the distal end of the radius and ulna.
Symptoms	Sudden pain; loss of function; direct and indirect tenderness.
Signs	Loss of function; possible deformity; rapid swelling; direct tenderness; indirect tenderness; possible bony deviation; possible crepitus; possible false joint motion; delayed ecchymosis; possible median nerve damage resulting from a fracture of the ulna and radius.
Special Tests	Not applicable
Referral/ Diagnostic Procedure	Refer to an orthopedist. X–ray.
Classification of Injury	Not applicable

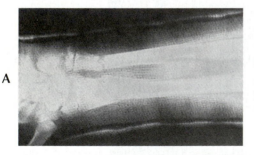
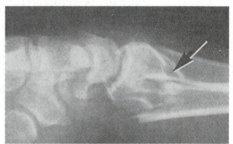

A   B

Colles' fracture, lateral view. The lateral view shows a fracture with comminuted fragments. The typical dorsal concave angulation is readily apparent *(arrow).*

Medical Term	Hamate fracture
Common Term	Same as above
Mechanisms	Indirect trauma to the wrist; a fall on an outstretched hand or hyperextended wrist.
Symptoms	Sudden pain; loss of function; direct and indirect tenderness.
Signs	Loss of function; possible deformity; rapid swelling; direct tenderness; indirect tenderness; possible bony deviation; possible crepitus; possible false motion; delayed ecchymosis.
Special Tests	Not applicable
Referral/ Diagnostic Procedure	Refer to an orthopedist. X–ray, CT scan.
Classification of Injury	Not applicable

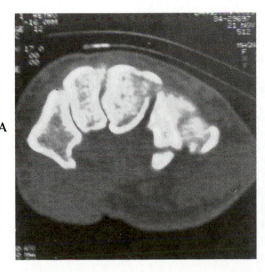 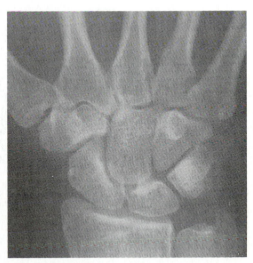

A, Hamate fracture, oblique view. Nondisplaced fracture of the medial aspect of the hamate bone is seen. **B**, Hamate fracture, oblique view.

Medical Term	**Lunate luxation**
Common Term	Dislocated carpal bone
Mechanisms	Indirect trauma; fall on an outstretched hand or a hyper-extended wrist.
Symptoms	Pain; loss of function; numbness of flexor muscles due to pressure on medial nerve; tenderness.
Signs	Marked deformity; loss of function; swelling; point tenderness; Murphy's sign.
Special Tests	Not applicable
Referral/ Diagnostic Procedure	Refer to an orthopedist. X–ray for possible fracture.
Classification of Injury	Not applicable

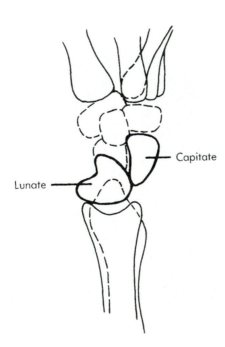

The lunate is rotated in a palmar direction and loses
its normal alignment to the distal radius.

Medical Term	**Wrist ganglion**
Common Term	Bible cyst
Mechanisms	Herniation resulting from minor dorsal or volar capsule sprains of the joint capsule through a process of mucoid degeneration or herniation of the synovial sheath of the flexor carpi radialis tendon sheath, the digital extensors, and the roof of the first dorsal compartment.
Symptoms	Pain; loss of function; discomfort on use of the hand and wrist.
Signs	Appears slowly after injury as a bump on the back of the wrist. It may appear, then disappear, then reappear.
Special Tests	Not applicable
Referral/ Diagnostic Procedure	Refer to an orthopedist. MRI.
Classification of Injury	Not applicable

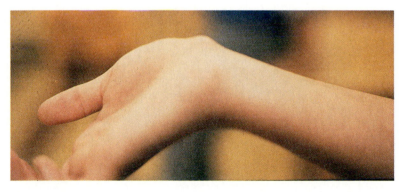

Wrist ganglion.

Medical Term	**Contusion of the wrist**
Common Term	Bruised wrist
Mechanisms	Direct trauma.
Symptoms	Pain; loss of function; transitory paralysis; tenderness.
Signs	Point tenderness; ecchymosis; hematoma formation; inflammation; loss of function.
Special Tests	Not applicable
Referral/ Diagnostic Procedure	Refer to a physician if symptoms/signs persist. X–ray.
Classification of Injury	First-, second-, and third-degree. See Chapter 1 for classification of contusion injury.

Medical Term	Carpal tunnel syndrome
Common Term	Same as above
Mechanisms	Compression of the median nerve as it passes beneath the flexor retinaculum on the volar aspect of the wrist.
Symptoms	Numbness and tingling in the fingers; pain; loss of function.
Signs	Point tenderness at the wrist; pain over the carpal tunnel; poor finger flexion.
Special Tests	Tinel's sign; Phalen's test. Electromyography; nerve conduction study.
Referral/ Diagnostic Procedure	Refer to an orthopedist. X–ray.
Classification of Injury	Not applicable

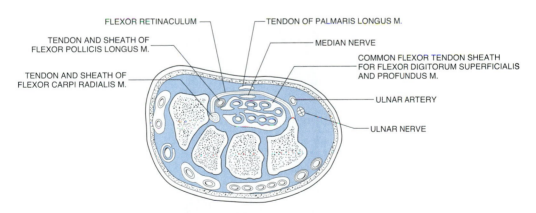

Cross-section of the right wrist. Note the carpal canal and the arrangement of the tendon sheaths.

Medical Term	**Distal radius and ulna epiphyseal plate injury**
Common Term	Fractured wrist
Mechanisms	Direct or indirect trauma from a fall on an outstretched hand or a hyperextended wrist.
Symptoms	Sudden pain; loss of function; direct and indirect tenderness.
Signs	Loss of function; possible deformity; rapid swelling; direct tenderness; indirect tenderness; possible bony deviation; possible crepitus; possible false motion; delayed ecchymosis.
Special Tests	Not applicable
Referral/ Diagnostic Procedure	Refer to an orthopedist. X–ray.
Classification of Injury	See Chapter 1 for classification of epiphyseal plate fractures.

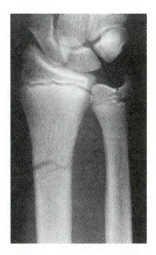

Closed reduction results in an anatomic reduction. Roentgenographic surveillance, however, is mandatory to ensure stability, because even minimal epiphyseal displacement requires prompt open reduction with internal fixation.

Medical Term	Forearm splints
Common Term	Same as above
Mechanisms	Static constant contraction of the forearm muscles causing minute tears in the interosseous membrane; overuse of muscles; irritation of the interosseous membrane and surrounding tissue.
Symptoms	Dull pain between the extensor muscles that cross the back of the forearm.
Signs	Pain on contraction of the extensor group of muscles; weakness of muscles against resistance; loss of function; inflammation.
Special Tests	Active and resistive movement; passive stretch.
Referral/ Diagnostic Procedure	Refer to an orthopedist. X–ray.
Classification of Injury	Not applicable

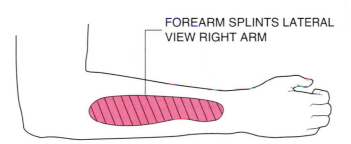

FOREARM SPLINTS LATERAL
VIEW RIGHT ARM

The shaded area of the right forearm denotes the area of possible pain for forearm splints.

Medical Term	**Distal radioulnar luxation**
Common Term	Dislocated wrist
Mechanisms	Indirect or direct trauma; forced hypersupination or hyperpronation of the forearm.
Symptoms	Pain on rotation of the wrist; loss of function.
Signs	Marked deformity; loss of function; swelling; point tenderness; increased prominence of the ulnar head; narrow wrist.
Special Tests	Not applicable
Referral/ Diagnostic Procedure	Refer to an orthopedist. X–ray for possible fracture.
Classification of Injury	Not applicable

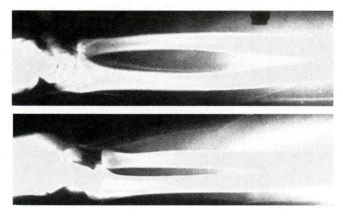

X-ray indication of a displaced distal ulna.

Medical Term	**Wrist luxation**
Common Term	Dislocated wrist
Mechanisms	Direct trauma causing hyperextension of the wrist.
Symptoms	Pain; loss of function.
Signs	Marked deformity; loss of function; swelling; point tenderness.
Special Tests	Not applicable
Referral/ Diagnostic Procedure	Refer to an orthopedist. X–ray for possible fracture.
Classification of Injury	Not applicable

Medical Term	Wrist sprain
Common Term	Same as above
Mechanisms	Overuse; stretching of the wrist ligaments due to a direct or indirect force applied to the joint as in axial loading, twisting, or impact.
Symptoms	Pain on active movement or passive stress of the joint; loss of function; pain on resistive movement; tenderness.
Signs	Point tenderness over the ligaments; swelling; hemorrhage; possible deformity with third-degree injury; ecchymosis; possible instability with second- and third-degree injury; inflammation.
Special Tests	Active and resistive movements; passive stress test.
Referral/ Diagnostic Procedure	Refer to an orthopedist if symptoms/signs persist.
Classification of Injury	First-, second-, and third-degree. See Chapter 1 for classification of sprain injury.

Medical Term	**Wrist strain**
Common Term	Same as above
Mechanisms	Trauma to the musculotendinous unit, due to excessive forcible contraction or stretching, and muscle fatigue.
Symptoms	Pain increased with active movement; pain on passive stretch; loss of function; possible snapping sound heard when injury occurs; muscle fatigue before injury occurs; pain on resistive movement, tenderness.
Signs	Muscle spasm; swelling; ecchymosis; point tenderness; loss of function; loss of strength; hematoma formation and defect in musculotendinous unit with third-degree injury; inflammation; possible calcium formation with third-degree injury.
Special Tests	Active and resistive movement; passive stretch.
Referral/ Diagnostic Procedure	Refer to an orthopedist if symptoms/signs persist.
Classification of Injury	First-, second-, and third-degree. See Chapter 1 for classification of strain injury.

■ TESTS FOR THE EVALUATION OF INJURIES TO THE ■ WRIST

■ GENERAL ASSESSMENT FOR JOINT RANGE OF MOTION AND STRENGTH FOR STRAIN, TENDINITIS, AND TENOSYNOVITIS

Active Movement

The athlete moves the body part through the range of motion actively, trying to reproduce the pain.

Passive Stretch

The athletic trainer performs a passive stretch of the involved muscle or tendon.

Resistive Movement

The athlete moves the body part through the range of motion, while the athletic trainer applies resistance.

■ GENERAL ASSESSMENT FOR JOINT RANGE OF MOTION AND LIGAMENTOUS STABILITY FOR A SPRAIN

Active Movement

The athlete moves the joint through the range of motion actively. The athletic trainer should be looking for any limitations in the range of motion.

Passive Movement

If the athlete cannot move the joint through the range of motion actively, then passive range of motion should be done to determine if the range of motion is blocked due to the athlete's pain, or if some obstacle is blocking the joint.

Resistive Movement

The athlete moves the joint through the range of motion, while the athletic trainer applies resistance.

Passive Stress

The athletic trainer applies stress to the joint to test the integrity of the ligamentous structures of the joint.

■ TEST FOR CARPAL TUNNEL SYNDROME

Phalen's Sign

The athlete flexes the wrists maximally and holds this position for 1 minute by pushing both the wrists together. A positive test indicates tingling that radiates into the thumb, index finger, and the middle and lateral half of the fourth finger.

Tinel's Sign

The athletic trainer taps over the volar carpal ligament. A positive test is indicated by a tingling sensation along the median nerve distribution.

■ TEST FOR VASCULAR OCCLUSION

Allen's test

The athletic trainer uses finger pressure to occlude the radial and ulnar arteries. The athlete opens and closes the fist several times to express any remaining blood. The athletic trainer releases the pressure one artery at a time. Negative sign if pale skin of the palm flushes immediately. Positive sign if skin remains pale for more than 5 seconds.

HAND INJURIES AND CONDITIONS

Chapter 9

Medical Term	**Mallet finger**
Common Term	Hammer finger
Mechanisms	Longitudinal force to the fingertip; forced flexion of the distal phalanx.
Symptoms	Pain; loss of function; inability to extend the distal phalanx.
Signs	Deformity; finger tip is dropped down; possible crepitus; inability to extend distal phalanx; finger carried at 30°.
Special Tests	Test for range of motion, extension, of the distal phalanx.
Referral/ Diagnostic Procedure	Refer to an orthopedist. X–ray for avulsion fracture.
Classification of Injury	Not applicable

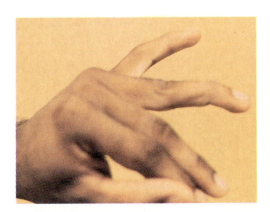 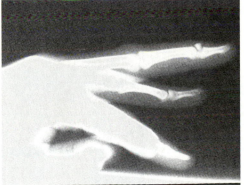

A, Mallet finger indicated by flexion of DIP joint. **B**, X-ray of an avulsion of the extensor tendon from its insertion, causing inability to extend the DIP joint.

Medical Term	**Boutonnière deformity**
Common Term	Buttonhole deformity
Mechanisms	Trauma to middle phalanx; forced flexion of the proximal interphalangeal joint. Rupture of the extensor tendon of the middle phalanx.
Symptoms	Pain at point of injury; loss of function.
Signs	Point tenderness over the middle phalanx (dorsum side); swelling; flexion deformity of the proximal interphalangeal joint; inability to extend the finger; hyperextension of the distal joint.
Special Tests	Range of motion of the PIP joint.
Referral/ Diagnostic Procedure	Refer to an orthopedist. X–ray for possible fracture.
Classification of Injury	Not applicable

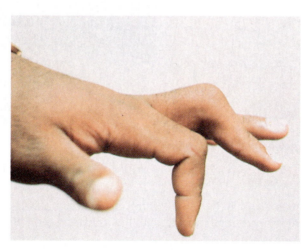

Boutonnière deformity caused by a rupture of the extensor tendon of the middle phalange.

Medical Term	**Bowler's hand**
Common Term	Bowler's thumb
Mechanisms	Overuse of the thumb, such as in the hole of a bowling ball, causing pressure on the ulnar nerve.
Symptoms	Numbness; pain; tingling.
Signs	Loss of sensation of the thumb; loss of strength.
Special Tests	Not applicable
Referral/ Diagnostic Procedure	Refer to a neurologist if symptoms/signs persist.
Classification of Injury	Not applicable

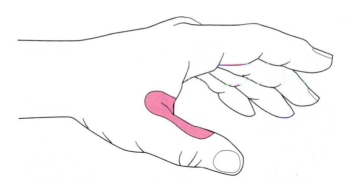

Area of pain for bowler's thumb (shaded area).

Medical Term	**Contusion of the hand**
Common Term	Bruise
Mechanisms	Direct trauma.
Symptoms	Pain; loss of function of the hand; transitory paralysis; tenderness.
Signs	Point tenderness; ecchymosis; hematoma formation; inflammation; loss of function.
Special Tests	Active, passive, and resistive range of motion of the hand.
Referral/ Diagnostic Procedure	Refer to an orthopedist if symptoms/signs persist. X–ray.
Classification of Injury	First-, second-, and third-degree. See Chapter 1 for classification of contusion injury.

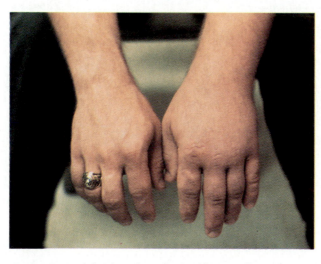

Contusion of the hand, indicated by swelling.

Medical Term	DeQuervain's disease
Common Term	Tenosynovitis of the wrist
Mechanisms	Extensive wrist motion, as in gripping sports, to the abductor pollicis longus and extensor pollicis brevis tendons and their sheaths at the radial styloid, excessive radial deviation; ulnar deviation; or a combination of these movements.
Symptoms	Aching; radiating pain into the hand and forearm; loss of strength; pain; inability to grip, point tenderness.
Signs	Painful crepitus of the tendon at the base of the thumb; weakness of thumb extension and abduction; paresthesia over the dorsum of the thumb; weakness in ulnar deviation; inflammation; possible stenosis of the fibroosseous canal; possible localized swelling.
Special Tests	Finkelstein's test.
Referral/ Diagnostic Procedure	Refer to orthopedist if symptoms/signs persist.
Classification of Injury	Not applicable

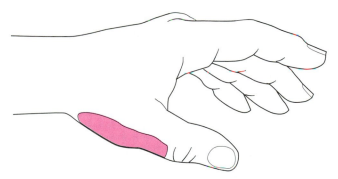

Area of pain for deQuervain's disease.

Medical Term	Felon
Common Term	Finger cellulitis
Mechanisms	Infection of the pulp of the finger tip, often caused by puncture wound.
Symptoms	Pain; throbbing.
Signs	Swelling; redness of the tip of the finger; inflammation.
Special Tests	Not applicable
Referral/ Diagnostic Procedure	Refer to a physician if signs/symptoms exist.
Classification of Injury	Not applicable

Medical Term	Barton's fracture
Common Term	Fracture of the distal radius
Mechanisms	Indirect trauma; a fall on an outstretched hand.
Symptoms	Sudden pain; loss of function; direct or indirect tenderness.
Signs	Loss of function; possible deformity; rapid swelling; direct or indirect tenderness; possible bony deviation; possible crepitus; possible false motion; delayed ecchymosis.
Special Tests	Not applicable
Referral/ Diagnostic Procedure	Refer to an orthopedist. X–ray.
Classification of Injury	Not applicable

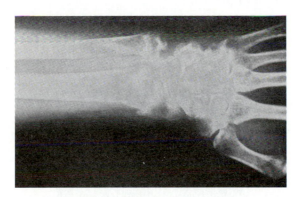

X-ray of a Barton's fracture at the distal radius.

Medical Term   Bennett's fracture

Common Term   Same as above

Mechanisms   Indirect trauma, such as striking an object with a closed fist on the first metacarpal.

Symptoms   Sudden pain; loss of function; direct or indirect tenderness.

Signs   Loss of function; possible deformity; rapid swelling; direct tenderness at the base of the first metacarpal; indirect tenderness; possible bony deviation; possible crepitus; possible false motion; delayed ecchymosis. The athlete may feel a click as the joint subluxes.

Special Tests   Not applicable

Referral/ Diagnostic Procedure   Refer to an orthopedist. X–ray.

Classification of Injury   Not applicable

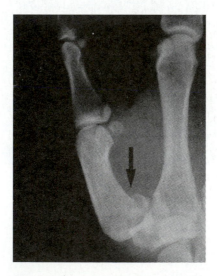

Bennett fracture, AP view *(arrow)*. Avulsion fracture of the articular surface of the first metacarpal, with subluxation at the carpometacarpal joint.

Medical Term   Fifth metacarpal fracture

Common Term   Boxer's fracture

Mechanisms   Indirect trauma, such as striking a blow with the fist.

Symptoms   Sudden pain; loss of function; direct or indirect tenderness; poor ability to grip.

Signs   Loss of function; inability to grip; rapid swelling; possible deformity; direct and indirect tenderness; possible bony deviation; possible crepitus; possible false motion; delayed ecchymosis.

Special Tests   Axial load test.

Referral/ Diagnostic Procedure   Refer to an orthopedist. X–ray.

Classification of Injury   Not applicable

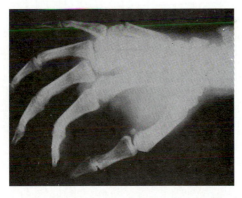

X-ray of fifth metacarpal fracture, called boxer's fracture.

Medical Term	**Carpal fracture**
Common Term	Same as above
Mechanisms	Direct trauma.
Symptoms	Sudden pain; loss of function; direct or indirect tenderness.
Signs	Loss of function; possible deformity; rapid swelling; direct or indirect tenderness; possible bony deviation; possible crepitus; possible false motion; delayed ecchymosis.
Special Tests	Not applicable
Referral/ Diagnostic Procedure	Refer to an orthopedist. X–ray.
Classification of Injury	Not applicable

Medical Term	**Metacarpal(s) fracture**
Common Term	Same as above
Mechanisms	Direct trauma.
Symptoms	Sudden pain; loss of function; direct or indirect tenderness.
Signs	Loss of function; possible deformity; rapid swelling; direct or indirect tenderness; possible bony deviation; possible crepitus; possible false motion; delayed ecchymosis.
Special Tests	Axial load test.
Referral/ Diagnostic Procedure	Refer to an orthopedist. X–ray.
Classification of Injury	Not applicable

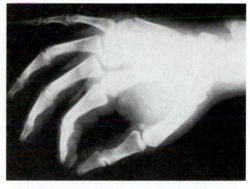

X-ray of a fractured phalange.

Medical Term	Phalanges fracture
Common Term	Same as above
Mechanisms	Indirect trauma; torsion to the end of the finger, longitudinal force applied to the tip of the finger.
Symptoms	Sudden pain; loss of function; direct and indirect tenderness.
Signs	Loss of function; possible deformity; rapid swelling; direct or indirect tenderness; possible bony deviation; possible crepitus; possible false motion; delayed ecchymosis.
Special Tests	Axial load test.
Referral/ Diagnostic Procedure	Refer to an orthopedist. X–ray.
Classification of Injury	Not applicable

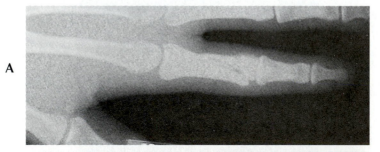

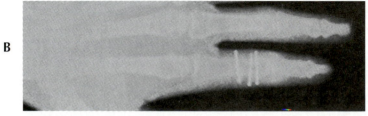

A, X-ray of a fractured phalange. **B**, Repair of a fractured phalange with pinning.

Medical Term	Smith's fracture
Common Term	Reverse Colles' fracture
Mechanisms	Direct trauma from a fall on the dorsum of the hand.
Symptoms	Sudden pain at the distal end of the radius and ulna; loss of function; direct or indirect tenderness.
Signs	Loss of function; possible deformity; rapid swelling; direct or indirect tenderness; possible bony deviation; possible crepitus; possible false motion; hand that is angled down; delayed ecchymosis.
Special Tests	Not applicable
Referral/ Diagnostic Procedure	Refer to an orthopedist. X–ray.
Classification of Injury	Not applicable

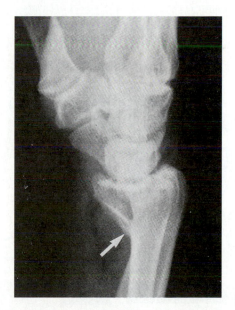

Smith fracture, lateral view. Note the volar displacement of the distal radius fragment *(arrow)*, giving the appearance of a reverse Colles' fracture.

Medical Term	**Phalange luxation (MPC, PIP, DIP)**
Common Term	Dislocated finger
Mechanisms	Direct trauma to the joint of a phalanx, indirect force applied to the distal tip of the finger.
Symptoms	Pain; loss of function.
Signs	Marked deformity; loss of function; swelling; point tenderness.
Special Tests	Not applicable
Referral/ Diagnostic Procedure	Refer to an orthopedist. X–ray for possible fracture.
Classification of Injury	Not applicable

A
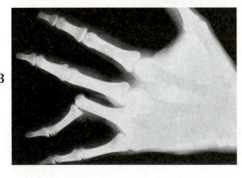

B
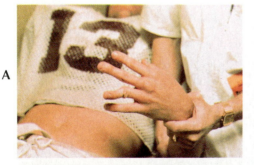

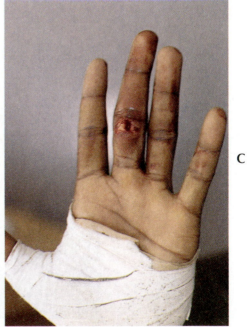
C

A, Phalange luxation. **B**, X-ray of luxation of the PIP joint. **C**, Open luxation of the PIP joint in a football player.

Medical Term	**Flexor digitorium profundus tendon rupture**
Common Term	Jersey finger
Mechanisms	Forced extension of flexed distal phalanx.
Symptoms	Pain; loss of function.
Signs	Swelling; loss of function; and pain that is distal to the interphalangeal (IP) joints and on the volar surface. The athletic trainer may palpate a mass on the palm of the hand of the tendon that was retracted. The athlete cannot fully flex the IP joints when the joint is held in extension.
Special Tests	Flexor digitorum profundus test.
Referral/ Diagnostic Procedure	Refer to an orthopedist.
Classification of Injury	Not applicable

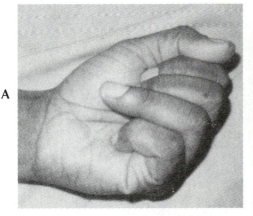 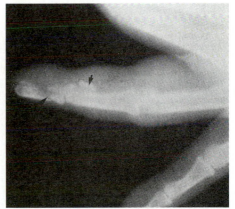

A   B

A, Rupture of the flexor profundus tendon, indicated by the athlete's ability to flex the DIP joint. **B**, X-ray showing an avulsion fracture of the flexor profundus tendon *(small arrow)* and fracture of the distal phalange *(large arrow)*.

Medical Term	**Finger collateral ligament sprain**
Common Term	Jammed finger
Mechanisms	Trauma; stretching of the ligament due to direct or indirect force applied to a joint.
Symptoms	Pain on active and resistive movements; pain on passive stress; loss of function; tenderness.
Signs	Point tenderness over ligament; swelling; hemorrhage; possible deformity with third-degree injury; ecchymosis; possible instability with second- and third-degree injury; inflammation.
Special Tests	Varus/valgus stress test, axial load test.
Referral/ Diagnostic Procedure	Refer to an orthopedist. X–ray for possible fracture.
Classification of Injury	First-, second-, and third-degree. See Chapter 1 for classification of sprain injury.

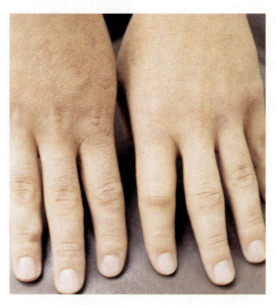

Swelling caused by a sprain of the collateral ligaments of the PIP joint.

Medical Term	**Ulnar collateral ligament of the thumb sprain**
Common Term	Gamekeeper's thumb; skier's thumb
Mechanisms	Forced abduction and hyperextension of the thumb causing sprain of the ulnar collateral ligament.
Symptoms	Pain on active and resistive movement; pain on passive stress; loss of function; tenderness.
Signs	Point tenderness over the ulnar collateral ligament; swelling; hemorrhage; possible deformity with third degree injury; instability with second- and third-degree injury; inflammation; pain on abduction of the thumb; ecchymosis.
Special Tests	Abduction stress test of the thumb.
Referral/ Diagnostic Procedure	Refer to an orthopedist. X–ray for possible avulsion fracture of ligament.
Classification of Injury	First-, second-, and third-degree. See Chapter 1 for classification of sprain injury.

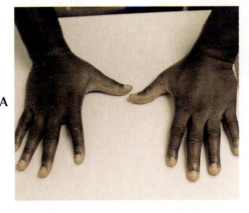 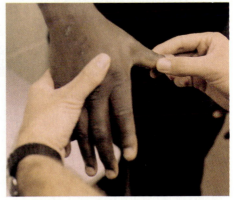

A B

A, Notice the abnormal abduction of the athlete's right thumb due to an ulnar collateral ligament injury of the metacarpophalangeal joint of the thumb.
B, Performing an abduction stress test of the injured thumb.

Medical Term	**Subungual hematoma**
Common Term	Blood under the nail
Mechanisms	Direct trauma to the fingernail.
Symptoms	Throbbing pain.
Signs	Blood can be seen under the nail.
Special Tests	Not applicable
Referral/ Diagnostic Procedure	Drill the nail to release the pressure and reduce the pain.
Classification of Injury	Not applicable

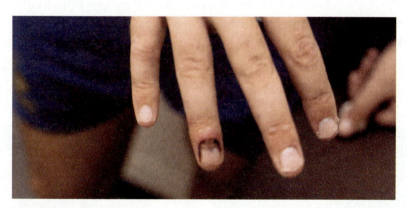

Subungual hematoma.

Medical Term	Tenosynovitis
Common Term	Same as above
Mechanisms	Overuse; direct trauma; repeated trauma.
Symptoms	Pain on active and resistive movement; pain on passive stretch; loss of function.
Signs	Swelling; thickened tendon in chronic cases; snowball crepitus; inflammation.
Special Tests	Active and resistive movement; passive stretch.
Referral/ Diagnostic Procedure	Refer to an orthopedist if symptoms/signs persist.
Classification of Injury	Not applicable

Medical Term	Ulnar neuropathy
Common Term	Handlebar palsy; cycle palsy
Mechanisms	Irritation of the ulnar nerve caused by abnormal pressure on the hands due to excessive body weight forced forward while the wrists are in prolonged extension; other causes are pressure on hypothenar eminence and road vibration during cycling.
Symptoms	Loss of strength; pain when riding; pain at rest; decrease in skin sensitivity; sharp burning pain.
Signs	Weakness of motor function; minimal sensory findings; loss of coordination of ulnar nerve in the fourth and fifth finger.
Special Tests	Motor test for ulnar nerve.
Referral/ Diagnostic Procedure	Refer to a neurologist. EMG study.
Classification of Injury	Not applicable

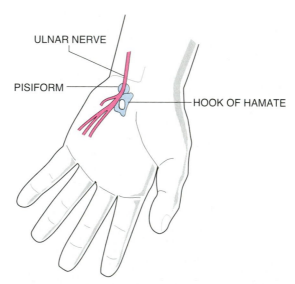

Pain and/or loss of sensation at the Tunnel of Guyon may indicate ulnar neuropathy. (The Tunnel of Guyon contains the ulnar nerve and artery.)

Medical Term	**Volar plate injury**
Common Term	Same as above
Mechanisms	Hyperextension of the proximal interphalangeal (PIP) joint.
Symptoms	Pain; loss of function.
Signs	Swelling; loss of function; possible subluxation of the joint; swan neck deformity.
Special Tests	Passive hyperextension compared to uninvolved PIP joint.
Referral/ Diagnostic Procedure	Refer to an orthopedist. X–ray for possible avulsion fracture.
Classification of Injury	Not applicable

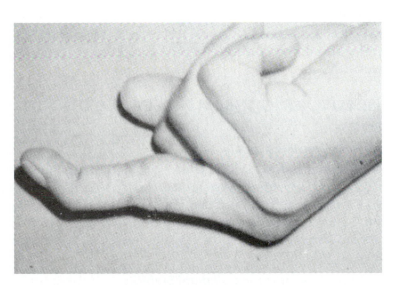

Volar instability of the PIP joint.

■ TESTS FOR THE EVALUATION OF INJURIES TO THE ■ HAND

Ulnar Nerve Test

Nerve	Ulnar
Sensation	Ulnar side of the hand, both dorsum and palm, lateral side of the fourth finger, and all of the fifth finger.
Sensation Test	Tip of the fifth finger, volar surface.
Motor Test	Adduction of the thumb against resistance; abduction of the index finger against resistance; adduction, and abduction against resistance, of the fourth and fifth fingers. Test adduction of the fourth and fifth fingers by placing a piece of paper between the fingers and trying to pull it out while the athlete tries to hold on to it.

■ TEST FOR DE QUERVAIN'S SYNDROME

Finkelstein's Test

The athletic trainer performs passive ulnar wrist deviation with the athlete's thumb flexed and adducted in the palm. Reproducing the athlete's pain if a positive test.

■ TEST FOR FLEXOR DIGITORUM PROFUNDUS TENDON RUPTURE

Flexor Digitorum Profundus Test

The athletic trainer holds the athlete's finger, stabilizing the metacarpophalangeal and interphalangeal joints in extension. The athletic trainer then asks the athlete to flex his distal interphalangeal joint. If the athlete can do this, the flexor digitorum profundus tendon is functional. If the athlete cannot perform the test, the tendon may be cut or the muscle denervated.

Valgus and Varus Stress Test for Collateral Stability

The athletic trainer applies an valgus and varus force to the joints of the finger to determine the stability of the joints. Looseness may indicate torn ligaments. There should be no motion in the metacarpophalangeal joint in flexion.

208

Abduction Stress Test of the Thumb for Ulnar Collateral Ligament

The athletic trainer applies an abduction stress to the thumb, testing for the integrity of the ulnar collateral ligament.

■ AXIAL LOAD TEST FOR BONY INTEGRITY

The athletic trainer compresses the bone from distal to proximal. Reproducing the athlete's pain is an indication for referral.

■ GENERAL ASSESSMENT OF JOINT RANGE OF MOTION AND STRENGTH FOR STRAIN, TENDINITIS, AND TENOSYNOVITIS

Active Movement

The athlete moves the body part through the range of motion actively, trying to reproduce the pain.

Passive Stretch

The athletic trainer performs a passive stretch of the involved muscle or tendon, trying to reproduce the pain.

Resistive Movement

The athlete moves the body part through the range of motion while the athletic trainer applies resistance, trying to reproduce the pain.

■ GENERAL ASSESSMENT OF JOINT RANGE OF MOTION AND LIGAMENTOUS STABILITY FOR A SPRAIN.

Active Movement

The athlete moves the joint through the range of motion actively, then passive range of motion should be done to determine if the range of motion is blocked due to the athlete's pain, or because some obstacle is blocking the joint.

Passive Movement

If the athlete cannot move the joint through the range of motion actively, then passive range of motion should be done to determine whether the range of motion is blocked due to the athlete's pain or because some object is blocking the joint.

Resistive Movement

If the athlete moves the joint through the range of motion, while the athletic trainer applies resistance, trying to reproduce the pain.

Passive Stress

The athletic trainer applies stress to the joint to test the integrity of the ligamentous structures of the joint.

THORACIC INJURIES AND CONDITIONS

Chapter 10

Medical Term	**Breast contusion**
Common Term	Jogger's breast
Mechanisms	Repetitive and excessive movement of the breast stretching Cooper's ligament in females.
Symptoms	Pain; tenderness.
Signs	Tenderness; ecchymosis; hematoma formation; inflammation.
Special Tests	Active, passive, resistive range of motion test.
Referral/ Diagnostic Procedure	Refer to a gynecologist or family practice physician if symptoms/signs persist.
Classification of Injury	First-, second-, and third-degree. See Chapter 1 for classification of contusion injury.

Medical Term	**Breast contusion**
Common Term	Bruised breast
Mechanisms	Direct trauma
Symptoms	Pain; tenderness.
Signs	Tenderness; ecchymosis; hematoma formation; inflammation.
Special Tests	Not applicable
Referral/ Diagnostic Procedure	Refer to a gynecologist or family practice physician if symptoms/signs persist.
Classification of Injury	First-, second-, and third-degree. See Chapter 1 for classification of contusion injury.

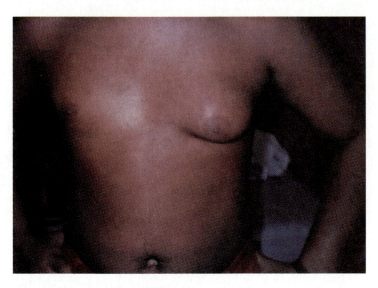

Breast contusion due to direct trauma.

Medical Term	**Celiac (solar) plexus syndrome**
Common Term	Wind knocked out
Mechanisms	Direct trauma to the celiac (solar) plexus by an external object causing paralysis of the diaphragm muscle.
Symptoms	Pain; trouble breathing normally.
Signs	Anoxia; inability to breathe normally; hysteria.
Special Tests	Not applicable
Referral/ Diagnostic Procedure	Not applicable
Classification of Injury	Not applicable

Medical Term	Rib contusion
Common Term	Bruised ribs
Mechanisms	Direct trauma to ribs.
Symptoms	Pain on breathing; loss of function; transitory paralysis of muscles involved with the rib cage; tenderness.
Signs	Point tenderness; loss of function; possible ecchymosis; hematoma formation; inflammation.
Special Tests	Not applicable
Referral/ Diagnostic Procedure	Refer to an orthopedist. X–ray for possible rib fracture.
Classification of Injury	First-, second-, and third-degree. See Chapter 1 for classification of contusion injury.

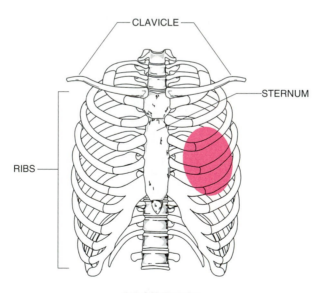

RIB CONTUSION

One possible area of pain from force *(shaded area)* directed to ribs.

Medical Term	Sternum contusion
Common Term	Bruised sternum
Mechanisms	Direct trauma to the sternum, such as a helmet to the ribs.
Symptoms	Pain over sternum; pain on breathing; tenderness over the sternum; pain on chest expansion.
Signs	Tenderness; possible ecchymosis; hematoma formation; inflammation.
Special Tests	Not applicable
Referral/ Diagnostic Procedure	Refer to an orthopedist or a cardiologist.
Classification of Injury	First-, second-, and third-degree. See Chapter 1 for classification of contusion injury.

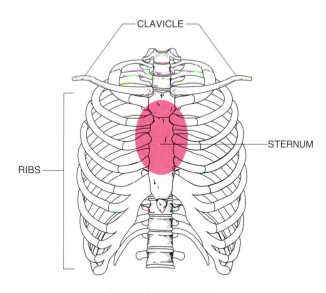

STERNUM CONTUSION

Painful portion of sterum and surrounding area from direct trauma (*shaded area*).

Medical Term	**Costochondral separation**
Common Term	Bruised ribs
Mechanisms	Direct or indirect trauma, depressing the rib cage.
Symptoms	Pain on movement of the thoracic area; difficulty breathing; loss of function; tenderness, popping sound heard at time of separation.
Signs	Swelling; point tenderness; possible deformity; loss of function.
Special Tests	Not applicable
Referral/ Diagnostic Procedure	Refer to an orthopedist. X–ray for possible rib fracture.
Classification of Injury	Not applicable

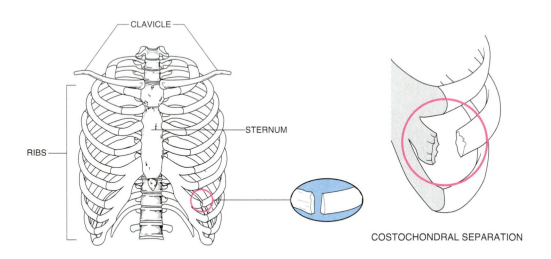

One possible articulation where costochondral separation could occur.

Medical Term	**Costovertebral joint sprain**
Common Term	Same as above
Mechanisms	Trauma; overuse; stretching of a costovertebral ligaments due to a direct or indirect force applied to a joint; compression of ribs; twisting of trunk.
Symptoms	Pain on active movement; pain on passive stress; loss of function of thoracic movement; pain on breathing; radiating pain on the side of injury; pain in the scapular area.
Signs	Point tenderness over the ligament; swelling; hemorrhage; possible deformity with third-degree injury; inflammation; pain on breathing.
Special Tests	Active and resistive movements; passive stress.
Referral/ Diagnostic Procedure	Refer to an orthopedist. X–ray for possible fracture.
Classification of Injury	First-, second-, and third-degree. See Chapter 1 for classification of sprain injury.

Medical Term	**Rib fracture**
Common Term	Broken rib
Mechanisms	Direct or indirect trauma to the ribs.
Symptoms	Sudden pain; difficulty breathing; direct and indirect tenderness.
Signs	Difficulty breathing; possible deformity; direct and indirect tenderness; possible bony deviations; possible crepitus; possible false motion; delayed ecchymosis.
Special Tests	Not applicable
Referral/ Diagnostic Procedure	Refer to an orthopedist. X–ray.
Classification of Injury	Not applicable

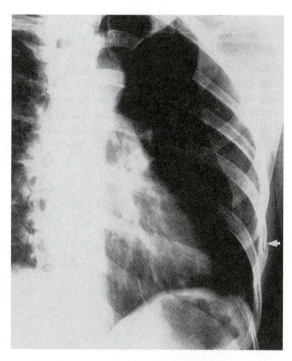

X-ray of fractured left sixth rib *(arrow)*.

Medical Term	**Sternum fracture**
Common Term	Broken sternum
Mechanisms	Direct trauma; posterior compression; hyperextension of the trunk.
Symptoms	Sudden pain; difficulty breathing; direct and indirect tenderness; sharp chest pain.
Signs	Difficulty breathing; rapid swelling; possible deformity; direct and indirect tenderness; possible bony deviation; possible crepitus; possible false motion; delayed ecchymosis.
Special Tests	Not applicable
Referral/ Diagnostic Procedure	Refer to an orthopedist and a cardiologist. X–ray.
Classification of Injury	Not applicable

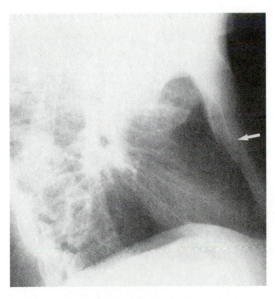

X-ray indicating lateral view of sternum.

Medical Term	**Jogger's nipple**
Common Term	Runner's nipple
Mechanisms	Friction caused by rubbing of clothing.
Symptoms	Irritation, pain at the nipple.
Signs	Possible bleeding and hardness.
Special Tests	Not applicable
Referral/ Diagnostic Procedure	Refer to a physician if symptoms/signs persist.
Classification of Injury	Not applicable

Medical Term	**Spontaneous pneumothorax**
Common Term	Collapsed lung
Mechanisms	The presence of air within the chest cavity in the pleural space outside the lung as a result of an indirect force trauma to the anterior, lateral, or posterior thoracic area. Usually in males between the ages of 20 and 40.
Symptoms	Sharp chest pain; difficulty breathing.
Signs	Respiratory distress.
Special Tests	Not applicable
Referral/ Diagnostic Procedure	Refer to a pulmonary specialist.
Classification of Injury	Not applicable

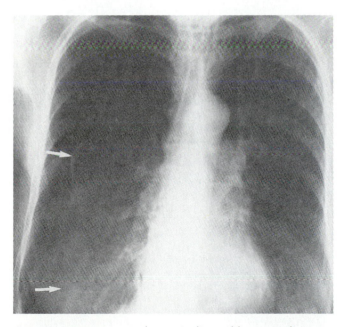

Spontaneous pneumothorax indicated by partial collapse of right lung *(arrows)*.

Medical Term	**Tension pneumothorax**
Common Term	Collapsed lung
Mechanisms	Direct trauma; lung punctured by rib; sucking wound; possibly preceded by spontaneous pneumothorax.
Symptoms	Pain; difficulty in breathing.
Signs	Respiratory distress; bulging tissue between ribs and above clavicle, distension of neck veins.
Special Tests	Not applicable
Referral/ Diagnostic Procedure	Refer to a pulmonary specialist.
Classification of Injury	Not applicable

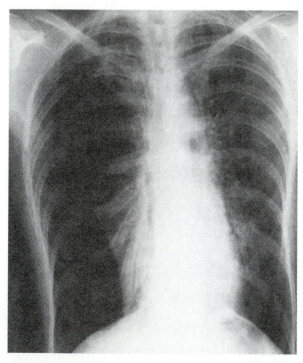

Right lung is collapsed, and there is a slight shift of the mediastinum to the left.

LOWER BACK INJURIES AND CONDITIONS

Chapter 11

Compression Fracture
Transverse Process Fracture
Lumbar Herniation/Intervertebral
  Disk Rupture
Nerve Root Compression
Sciatica
Spondylitis

Spondylolisthesis
Spondylolysis
Spondylosis
Intervertebral Sprain
Lumbosacral Sprain
Sacroiliac Sprain
Lumbosacral Strain

Medical Term	**Compression fracture**
Common Term	Same as above
Mechanisms	Forced flexion of the spine.
Symptoms	Sudden pain; loss of the range of motion of the spine; direct and indirect tenderness over the vertebral column; numbness—unilateral or bilateral.
Signs	Loss of range of motion of the spine; direct tenderness; indirect tenderness; possible crepitus; possible numbness in area of the associated dermatome; pain that increases with movement.
Special Tests	Not applicable
Referral/ Diagnostic Procedure	Refer to an orthopedic surgeon. X–ray.
Classification of Injury	See Chapter 1 for fracture.

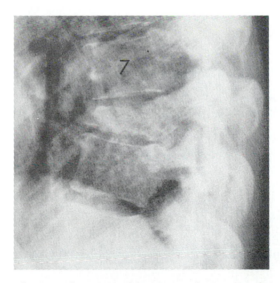

Thoracic fracture subluxation of T8. Lateral radiograph shows the compression of T8. (T7 shown here marked as 7.)

Medical Term	**Transverse process fracture**
Common Term	Same as above
Mechanisms	Direct trauma to the vertebrae; indirect trauma as in a violent torsion movement.
Symptoms	Sudden pain; loss of range of motion of the spine; direct or indirect tenderness.
Signs	Loss of range of motion of the spine; rapid swelling; direct tenderness; indirect tenderness; possible bony deviation; possible crepitus; possible false joint motion.
Special Tests	Not applicable
Referral/ Diagnostic Procedure	Refer to an orthopedic surgeon. X–ray.
Classification of Injury	See Chapter 1 for fracture.

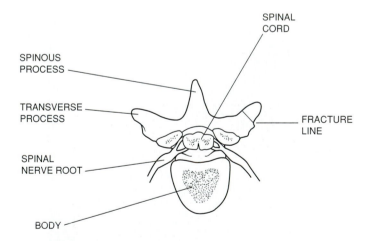

Location of fracture of transverse process lateral to vertebral body.

Medical Term	**Lumbar herniation/Intervertebral disk rupture**
Common Term	Slipped disk
Mechanisms	Trauma; abnormal stress due to faulty body mechanics, as in a twisting motion or lifting.
Symptoms	Pain and point tenderness in the lumbar region; pain on nerve distribution that increases with coughing or sneezing; numbness; muscle weakness.
Signs	Painful arch; the athlete will tilt away from the side of injury on flexion and extension; possible sensory loss in dermatomes; absent or decreased reflexes (achilles and patella); possible weakness of foot dorsiflexors and inversion.
Special Tests	Straight leg raise; well leg/straight leg raise test; Hoover test; Kernig test; Milgram test; Naffziger test; Valsalva test; general assessment of lumbar range of motion and strength test and neurologic evaluation.
Referral/ Diagnostic Procedure	Refer to a neurosurgeon. X–ray, MRI.
Classification of Injury	Not applicable

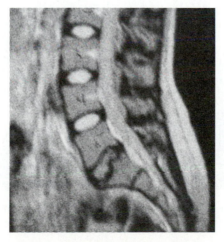

MRI of a herniation of L5 disk.

Medical Term	**Nerve root compression**
Common Term	Compressed nerve
Mechanisms	Trauma.
Symptoms	Numbness; paresthesia; pain; loss of function, tenderness.
Signs	Loss of range of normal spinal range of motion, decreased sensation in one or more dermatomes; muscle weakness; absent or decreased reflexes.
Special Tests	Straight leg raise; well leg/straight leg raise test; Hoover test; Kernig test; Milgram test; Naffziger test; Valsalva test; general assessment of spinal range of motion and strength test, and neurologic evaluation assessment.
Referral/ Diagnostic Procedure	Refer to a neurosurgeon. X–ray, MRI.
Classification of Injury	Not applicable

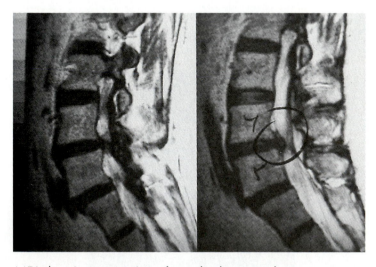

MRI showing narrowing of vertebral spaces due to compression of disk.

Medical Term	Sciatica
Common Term	Not applicable
Mechanisms	Nerve compression from disk lesion.
Symptoms	Radiating pain on nerve pathway; paresthesia.
Signs	Loss of function of the lumbar spine; positive well straight leg raising test; positive straight leg raising test, muscle spasm.
Special Tests	Well leg/straight leg raise test; straight leg raise test; Hoover test; Kernig test; assessment of range of motion and strength test, and lumbar spine neurologic evaluation.
Referral/ Diagnostic Procedure	Refer to an orthopedic surgeon or neurosurgeon.
Classification of Injury	Not applicable

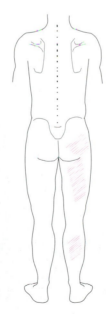

Areas of referred pain
from sciatica.

Medical Term	**Spondylitis**
Common Term	Backache
Mechanisms	Unknown. The course of the condition is slow and variable over a 10- to 20-year period.
Symptoms	Pain longer than 3 months in duration; stiffness that can affect the sacroiliac joint; radiating pain in one or both legs.
Signs	Gradual limitations of range of motion; tenderness in the sacroiliac joint; as the condition progresses, x–ray will demonstrate widespread bridging of the vertebrae by desmophytes referred to as "Bamboo Spine."
Special Tests	Gaenslen's sign; pelvic rock test; Fabere test; range of motion and neurological evaluation.
Referral/ Diagnostic Procedure	Refer to an orthopedic surgeon. X–ray.
Classification of Injury	Not applicable

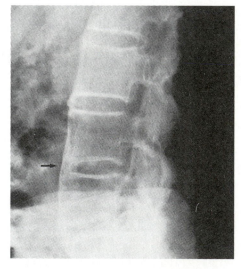

Lateral x-ray of the lumbar spine showing syndesmorphytes (calcification of ligament) characteristic of ankylosing spondylitis *(arrow)*.

Medical Term	Spondylolisthesis
Common Term	Backache
Mechanisms	Direct trauma; spondylolysis or congenital deformity.
Symptoms	Chronic backache; possible sciatica; increase in pain from standing and after activity; possible radiating pain in legs and buttocks.
Signs	Forward slippage of vertebrae, usually L5 on S1; increased lordosis.
Special Tests	Straight leg raise test; well leg/straight leg raise test; Hoover test; Kernig test; assessment of range of motion, and neurologic evaluation.
Referral/ Diagnostic Procedure	Refer to an orthopedic surgeon. X–ray.
Classification of Injury	Not applicable

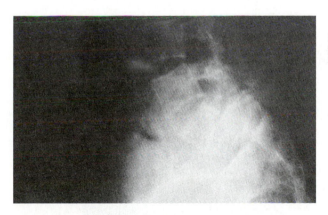

Lateral x-ray showing displacement of L5 on S1, indicating spondylolithesis.

Medical Term	**Spondylolysis**
Common Term	Backache
Mechanisms	Degeneration of lumbar vertebrae; common to gymnasts and football linemen. It is caused by a congenital or acquired defect in the pars interarticularis and/or repeated trauma to the area of affected vertebrae.
Symptoms	Back pain; loss of spinal range of motion; symptoms increase with weight bearing, and hyperextension causes pain.
Signs	X–ray demonstrates a defect in the neural arch, and a bone scan may show a hot spot.
Special Tests	Assessment of range of motion and neurologic evaluation.
Referral/ Diagnostic Procedure	Refer to an orthopedic surgeon. X–ray, bone scan.
Classification of Injury	Not applicable

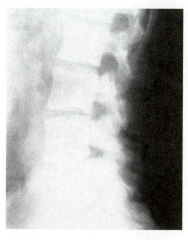

Lateral x-ray showing defect
in the pars interarticularis
indicative of spondylolysis
(scotty dog deformity).

Medical Term	Spondylosis
Common Term	Backache
Mechanisms	Repeated minor trauma; disk trauma due to incident; changes in lumbar vertebral body's interspaces related to chronic discopathy.
Symptoms	Increased back pain with activity; possible radiating pain; loss of function; pain on hyperextension.
Signs	Possible hypalgesia; loss of function. X–ray may show narrowing of intervertebral space.
Special Tests	Straight leg raise test; well leg/straight leg raise test; hyperextension test; Hoover test; Kernig test; Milgram test; Naffziger test; Valsalva test; assessment of spinal range of motion and neurologic evaluation.
Referral/ Diagnostic Procedure	Refer to an orthopedic surgeon. X–ray, myelogram.
Classification of Injury	Not applicable

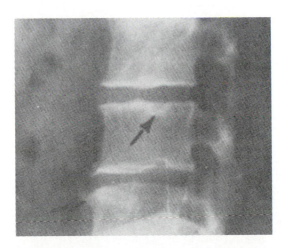

Lateral x-ray of degenerative changes at the L2/L3/L4 and L4/L5 level causing disk space narrowing *(arrow)*.

Medical Term	Intervertebral sprain
Common Term	Backache
Mechanisms	Trauma; overuse; stretching of a ligament due to direct or indirect force applied to a joint.
Symptoms	Pain on active movement of the affected area of the spine; pain on passive stress; loss of function; pain on resistive movement; tenderness.
Signs	Point tenderness over ligament; swelling; hemorrhage; possible deformity with third-degree injury; ecchymosis; inflammation; loss of function.
Special Tests	Assessment of range of motion and ligamentous stability.
Referral/ Diagnostic Procedure	Refer to an orthopedic surgeon if symptoms/signs persist.
Classification of Injury	First-, second-, and third-degree. See Chapter 1 for classification of sprain.

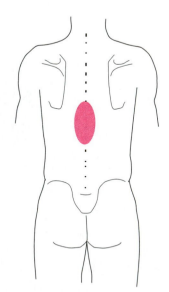

Area of pain for intervertebral sprain.

Medical Term	Lumbosacral sprain
Common Term	Low back sprain
Mechanisms	Trauma; overuse; stretching of a ligament due to a direct or indirect force applied to a joint.
Symptoms	Pain on active movement; pain on passive stress; loss of function; pain on resistive movement; tenderness.
Signs	Point tenderness over the ligament; swelling; hemorrhage; possible deformity with third-degree injury; ecchymosis; inflammation; loss of range of motion of the lower back; on pelvis may be higher than the opposite side.
Special Tests	Assessment of range of motion and ligamentous stability.
Referral/ Diagnostic Procedure	Refer to an orthopedic surgeon if symptoms/signs persist.
Classification of Injury	First-, second-, and third-degree. See Chapter 1 for classification of sprain.

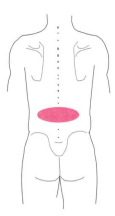

Area of pain for lumbrosacral sprain.

Medical Term	Sacroiliac sprain
Common Term	Backache
Mechanisms	Trauma; overuse; stretching of a ligament due to a direct or indirect force applied to a joint; abnormal posture.
Symptoms	Pain on active movement as in knee to chest movement; pain on passive stress; loss of function; tenderness; pain on resistive movement.
Signs	Point tenderness over the sacroiliac ligament; swelling; hemorrhage; possible deformity with third-degree injury; ecchymosis; inflammation; pain on knee to chest movement.
Special Tests	Pelvic rock; Fabere test; Gaenslen's test; assessment of range of motion and ligamentous stability.
Referral/ Diagnostic Procedure	Refer to an orthopedic surgeon is symptoms/signs persist.
Classification of Injury	First-, second-, and third-degree. See Chapter 1 for classification of sprain.

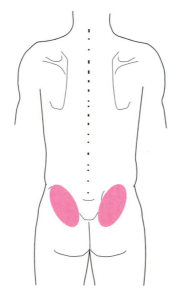

Areas of pain in sacroiliac sprain.

Medical Term	**Lumbosacral strain**
Common Term	Low back strain
Mechanisms	Trauma to the musculotendinous unit due to excessive forcible contraction or stretching and muscle fatigue.
Symptoms	Pain that increases with active movement, pain on passive stretch; loss of function; possible snapping sound heard when injury occurs; muscle fatigue before injury; pain on resistive movement; tenderness.
Signs	Muscle spasm; swelling; ecchymosis; point tenderness; loss of function; loss of strength; hematoma formation and defect in musculotendinous unit with third-degree injury; inflammation.
Special Tests	Pelvic rock test; Fabere test; Gaenslen's test; assessment of range of motion and strength test.
Referral/ Diagnostic Procedure	Refer to an orthopedic surgeon if symptoms/signs persist.
Classification of Injury	First-, second-, and third-degree. See Chapter 1 for classification of strain.

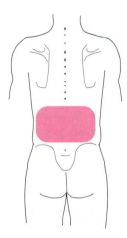

Area of pain for lumbrosacral strain.

■ TESTS FOR THE EVALUATION OF THE LOWER BACK ■

■ TESTS TO STRETCH THE SCIATIC NERVE OR SPINAL CORD

Straight Leg Raise Test

The athlete lies supine on a table, and the athletic trainer lifts the leg on the affected side of the body (keeping the leg straight) to approximately 80° of hip flexion. When the athlete experiences pain, the leg should be lowered slightly and the athlete asked to dorsiflex the ankle to see whether the pain is reproduced. If the pain is not reproduced, the pain is probably due to hamstring tightness. If the pain is reproduced with dorsiflexion, the athlete should be asked to point to the area of pain. This pain is probably due to sciatic nerve injury.

Well Leg / Straight Leg Raise Test

The athlete lies supine on a table, and the athletic trainer raises the unaffected leg in the same manner as the straight leg raise test. If this produces pain on the opposite side, this is further evidence that there is a space–occupying lesion causing pressure on the sciatic nerve.

Hoover Test

This is also called a malingering test. This test helps the athletic trainer decide if the athlete cannot raise the leg. The athletic trainer holds the athlete's heel of the uninvolved leg in the palm of the hand, then asks the athlete to perform a straight leg raise of the involved leg. The athletic trainer should feel a downward pressure in the palm of the hand if the athlete is really trying to raise the injured leg.

Kernig Test

The athlete lies supine on a table, places both hands behind the head and forcefully flexes the neck. Pain may be reproduced in the cervical or low back region. This indicates meningeal irritation or nerve root involvement.

■ TESTS TO INCREASE INTRATHECAL PRESSURE

Milgram Test

The athlete lies supine on a table, raises both legs approximately 2 to 3 inches (6 to 9 cm) off the table, while keeping the legs straight. The athlete is told to hold this position as long as possible without lowering the legs. If the athlete cannot hold this position for more than 30 seconds, there may be intrathecal or extrathecal pathology, such as a herniated disk.

Naffziger Test

The athlete lies supine on a table while the athletic trainer compresses the jugular veins for approximately 10 seconds. The athletic trainer then asks the athlete to cough. If this reproduces the pain, there is probably pressure on the theca.

Valsalva Test

The athlete is in the sitting position and is asked to bear down as if trying to have a bowel movement. If this causes pain, there is intrathecal pressure or injury involving the theca.

■ TESTS FOR THE SACROILIAC JOINT

Pelvic Rock Test

The athlete lies supine on a table, and the athletic trainer places the hands on the iliac crest with the thumbs on the anterior iliac spines. The athletic trainer then pushes his or her hands posterior toward the midline of the body, compressing the sacroiliac joint. If this produces pain, the sacroiliac joint may be injured.

Gaenslen's Test

The athlete lies supine on a table with the knees flexed to the chest. The athlete moves over to the edge of the table and slides one side of the buttocks off the table, then drops that leg off the table while keeping the other knee flexed to the chest. If this causes pain, then there may be injury to the sacroiliac joint.

Fabere Test

The athlete lies supine on a table and places the foot of the injured leg on the knee of the uninjured leg, placing the involved leg in a position of hip flexion, hip abduction, and external rotation. The athletic trainer then applies pressure to the knee of the injured leg, while applying pressure to the opposite anterior iliac spine, pushing in the opposite direction. If this causes pain, there may be injury to the sacroiliac joint.

■ RANGE OF MOTION TESTS *(All range of motion tests should be done actively, passively, and against resistance.)*

Painful Arc Test

The athletic trainer asks the athlete to flex as far as possible (touch the toes) and then extend as far as possible. The athletic trainer should ask the athlete where in the arc he or she is experiencing pain, and watch to see if the athlete is leaning to one side or the other when flexing and extending. Movement away from the side of the pain possibly indicates a disk lesion, and leaning toward the side of the injury possibly indicates a muscle spasm problem.

Lateral Bending Test

The athletic trainer should stabilize the hips of the athlete and ask him or her to lean to the left and then to the right. Pain while toward the side of the pain possibly indicates a disk lesion, and pain when leaning away from the side of the pain possibly indicates a muscle spasm problem.

Rotation Test

The athletic trainer places one hand on the shoulder of the athlete and the opposite hand on the iliac crest. The athlete is then asked to turn to the left and then to the right after the athletic trainer has changed hand position. Pain while rotating toward the side of the pain possibly indicates a disk lesion, and pain while rotating away from the side of the pain may indicate a muscle spasm problem.

■ NEUROLOGIC TESTS *(Neurologic tests will test muscles, reflexes, and sensory areas.)*

Nerve	**T12, L1, L2, L3**
Muscle	Iliopsoas
Test	Ask the athlete to flex the hip against resistance.
Reflex	None
Sensory	General thigh between the inguinal ligament and knee joint.
Nerve	**L2, L3, L4**
Muscle	Quadriceps and hip adductors
Test	Ask the athlete to extend the knee against resistance and adduct the hip against resistance.
Reflex	None
Sensory	General thigh and medial side of the leg.
Nerve	**L4**
Muscle	Tibialis anterior
Test	Ask the athlete to dorsiflex and invert the ankle against resistance.
Reflex	Patellar reflex
Sensory	Medial side of the leg.

Nerve	**L5**
Muscle	Extensor hallucis longus; gluteus medius; extensor digitorum longus.
Test	Ask the athlete to extend the great toe against resistance (extensor hallucis longus); have the athlete lie on the side and abduct the hip, or try to push the hip into adduction while the athlete resists (gluteus medius); and have the athlete extend the toes against resistance.
Reflex	None
Sensory	Lateral leg and dorsum of the foot.
Nerve	**S1**
Muscle	Peroneus longus and brevis; gastrocnemius/soleus; gluteus maximus.
Test	Ask the athlete to evert and dorsiflex the foot against resistance (peroneus longus and brevis); ask the athlete to plantar flex the ankle against resistance (gastrocnemius/soleus); ask the athlete to lie on a table with the knees flexed and the hip extended. Apply a downward force against the posterior thigh (gluteus maximus).
Reflex	Achilles tendon
Sensory	Lateral malleolus; lateral side and plantar surface of the foot.

■ PATHOLOGIC REFLEXES *(Presence of pathologic reflex indicates an upper motor neuron lesion, such as in a head injury.)*

Babinski Test

The athletic trainer draws a blunt object along the skin from the calcaneus up the foot to the toes. The toes should all flex at once. If the athlete has an expanding brain lesion, the great toe will extend and the other four toes will flex and spread apart.

Oppenheim Test

The athletic trainer draws a blunt object along the skin up the crest of the tibia. There should be no reaction or a reaction of pain. Athletes with a problem will have the same signs as with the Babinski test.

■ GENERAL ASSESSMENT TEST FOR RANGE OF MOTION AND STRENGTH FOR A STRAIN, TENDINITIS, AND TENOSYNOVITIS

Active Movement

The athlete moves the body part through the range of motion actively, trying to reproduce the pain.

Passive Stretch

The athletic trainer performs a passive stretch of the involved muscle or tendon.

Resistive Movement

The athlete moves the body part through the range of motion while the athletic trainer applies resistance.

■ GENERAL ASSESSMENT TEST FOR RANGE OF MOTION AND LIGAMENTOUS STABILITY FOR A SPRAIN

Active Movement

The athlete moves the joint through the range of motion actively. The athletic trainer should be looking for any limitations in the range of motion.

Passive Movement

If the athlete cannot move the joint through the range of motion actively, then passive range of motion should be done to determine if the range of motion is blocked due to the athlete's pain, or if some object is blocking the joint.

Resistive Movement

The athlete moves the joint through the range of motion while the athletic trainer applies resistance.

Passive Stress

The athletic trainer applies stress to the joint to test the integrity of the ligamentous structures of the joint.

ABDOMINAL INJURIES AND CONDITIONS

Chapter 12

Abdominal Muscle Contusion
Bladder Contusion
Kidney Contusion
Liver Contusion
Scrotal Contusion
Spleen Contusion
Abdominal Muscle Strain
Femoral Hernia

Inguinal Hernia
Kidney Laceration
Peritonitis
Spermatic Cord Torsion
Spleen Laceration
Stitch in the Side
Peptic Ulcer

Medical Term	**Abdominal muscle contusion**
Common Term	Bruised abdominal
Mechanisms	Direct trauma to abdominal muscles
Symptoms	Pain; loss of function; tightness in the abdominal area; tenderness.
Signs	Tightness in the abdominal area; tenderness; ecchymosis; hematoma formation; inflammation; loss of function; pain on sit–up test.
Special Tests	Sit–up test.
Referral/ Diagnostic Procedure	Refer to a physician if symptoms/signs persist.
Classification of Injury	First-, second-, and third-degree. See Chapter 1 for classification of contusion injury.

Medical Term	**Bladder contusion**
Common Term	Bruised bladder
Mechanisms	Direct trauma; long-distance running.
Symptoms	Pain in lower abdominal area; nausea; tenderness.
Signs	Referred pain in lower trunk; rigidity of abdominal muscles; possible vomiting; blood dripping from urethra; abdominal tenderness.
Special Tests	Not applicable
Referral/ Diagnostic Procedure	Refer the athlete to a physician.
Classification of Injury	First-, second-, and third-degree. See Chapter 1 for classification of contusion injury.

Medical Term	Kidney contusion
Common Term	Bruised kidney
Mechanisms	Direct contact; fall.
Symptoms	Pain; nausea.
Signs	Possible shock; possible vomiting; muscle spasm in back muscles; possible blood in urine (hematuria); referred pain in costovertebral area and lower abdominal area.
Special Tests	Not applicable
Referral/ Diagnostic Procedure	Refer to a nephrologist or a urologist. X–ray because the injury can be associated with a rib fracture.
Classification of Injury	Not applicable

Medical Term	Liver contusion
Common Term	Bruised liver
Mechanisms	Direct trauma to the right side of the rib cage.
Symptoms	Referred pain to the right scapula, shoulder, substernal area; possible pain in the left side of the chest; nausea.
Signs	Tenderness; inflammation; possible lower blood pressure and elevated pulse; possible nausea or vomiting; shock; worsening signs could mean laceration.
Special Tests	Monitor pulse and blood pressure.
Referral/ Diagnostic Procedure	Refer to a general surgeon. Hepatitis test.
Classification of Injury	Not applicable

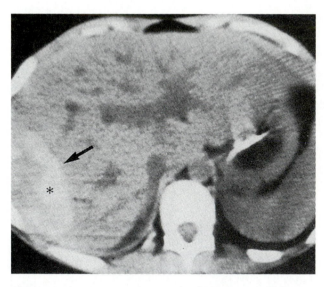

CT scan showing a subcapsular hematoma of the liver (*arrow*).

Medical Term	Scrotal contusion
Common Term	Not applicable
Mechanisms	Direct trauma.
Symptoms	Pain; nausea.
Signs	Swelling; ecchymosis; possible vomiting.
Special Tests	Not applicable
Referral/ Diagnostic Procedure	Refer to a physician if symptoms/signs persist.
Classification of Injury	Not applicable

Medical Term	**Spleen contusion**
Common Term	Same as above
Mechanisms	Direct trauma to the upper left quadrant of the abdominal area. If the trauma is severe enough, it can lead to a ruptured spleen.
Symptoms	Pain; nausea; possible referred pain in the left shoulder and arm (called a Kehr's sign); tenderness; recent history of mononucleosis.
Signs	Possible shock; rigidity in the upper left abdominal area; tachycardia; vomiting; possible loss of balance; tenderness.
Special Tests	Look for Kehr's sign; use Romberg test to check balance.
Referral/ Diagnostic Procedure	Refer to a general surgeon—medical emergency.
Classification of Injury	Not applicable

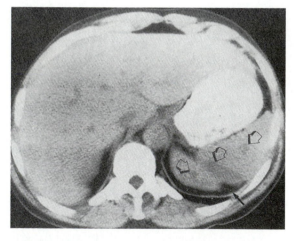

CT scan indicating multiple contusions (*open arrows*) to the spleen. Congenital defect (*closed arrow*) could be misinterpreted as the injury.

Medical Term	**Abdominal muscle strain**
Common Term	Pulled abdominal muscle
Mechanisms	Trauma to the musculotendinous unit due to excessive forcible contraction or stretching.
Symptoms	Pain increased on active movement; pain on passive stretch; loss of normal muscle function; tenderness.
Signs	Muscle spasm; swelling; ecchymosis; point tenderness; loss of strength; hematoma formation and defect in musculotendinous unit with third-degree injury; inflammation.
Special Tests	Assessment of range of motion and strength (sit–up).
Referral/ Diagnostic Procedure	Refer to a physician if symptoms/signs persist.
Classification of Injury	First-, second-, and third-degree. See Chapter 1 for classification of strain injury.

Medical Term	**Femoral hernia**
Common Term	Hernia
Mechanisms	Congenital or acquired through natural weakness, indirect trauma as in excessive strain. The hernia arises in the canal that transports the vessels and nerves to the leg.
Symptoms	A feeling of weakness; pulling sensation or pain in the groin area.
Signs	A protrusion in the groin area that is increased by coughing; point tenderness in the area of the hernia. Externally, looks like an inguinal hernia.
Special Tests	Coughing test.
Referral/ Diagnostic Procedure	Refer to a general surgeon.
Classification of Injury	Not applicable

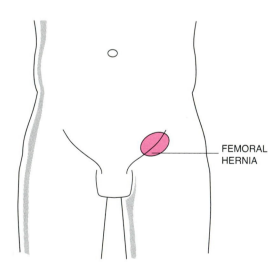

Area of possible protrusion and pain *(shaded area)* can occur on either side.

Medical Term	**Inguinal hernia**
Common Term	Hernia
Mechanisms	Congenital or acquired through natural weakness, direct trauma, or indirect trauma as in excessive strain. The hernia is located in the inguinal canal. Most common in males.
Symptoms	Weakness; pulling sensation or pain in the groin area.
Signs	A protrusion in the groin area that is increased by coughing. Externally, looks like a femoral hernia.
Special Tests	Coughing test.
Referral/ Diagnostic Procedure	Refer to a general surgeon.
Classification of Injury	Not applicable

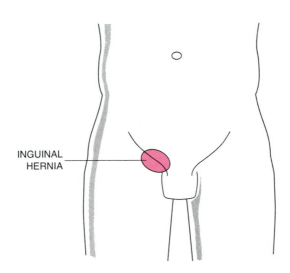

Area of possible protrusion and pain
(shaded area) can occur on either side.

Medical Term	**Kidney laceration**
Common Term	Same as above
Mechanisms	Direct trauma; congenital abnormality; violent muscle action.
Symptoms	Pain; nausea.
Signs	Shock; change in blood pressure and pulse; tenderness; muscle spasm; vomiting; referred pain in costovertebral area and lower abdominal area; blood in the urine (hematuria).
Special Tests	Not applicable
Referral/ Diagnostic Procedure	Refer to a physician.
Classification of Injury	Not applicable

Medical Term	**Peritonitis**
Common Term	Not applicable
Mechanisms	Inflammation caused by infection or trauma to peritoneum. Peritonitis can involve the stomach or the appendix.
Symptoms	Chills; fever to 102° F (39° C); nausea; pain; tenderness.
Signs	Positive rebound test; vomiting; diarrhea; abdominal tenderness; rapid breathing and pulse; tenderness; athlete lying on back with the thighs flexed.
Special Tests	Rebound test. (Athletic trainer applies pressure to athlete's abdominal area with hands, then releases pressure. Pain indicates positive test.)
Referral/ Diagnostic Procedure	Refer to a general surgeon.
Classification of Injury	Not applicable

Medical Term	**Spermatic cord torsion**
Common Term	Same as above
Mechanisms	Abnormal mobility of testicle; direct trauma.
Symptoms	Pain; nausea; a heavy feeling in the scrotum.
Signs	Swelling; tenderness; inflammation; possible vomiting.
Special Tests	Not applicable
Referral/ Diagnostic Procedure	Refer to a physician.
Classification of Injury	Not applicable

Medical Term	**Spleen laceration**
Common Term	Ruptured spleen
Mechanisms	Direct trauma to the upper left quadrant of the abdominal area.
Symptoms	Pain; nausea; referred pain in the left shoulder and arm (Kehr's sign); tenderness; recent history of mononucleosis.
Signs	Possible shock; abdominal rigidity; vomiting; tenderness.
Special Tests	Kehr's sign. Remember that the spleen can splint itself and break open at a later time.
Referral/ Diagnostic Procedure	Refer to a general surgeon—medical emergency.
Classification of Injury	Not applicable

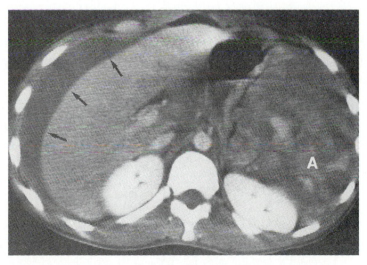

CT scan indicating disruption of the spleen after blunt abdominal trauma *(A)*. Arrows indicate a hemoperioneum.

Medical Term	Stitch in the side
Common Term	Same as above
Mechanisms	Varying causes: constipation; intestinal gas; poor conditioning; overeating.
Symptoms	Cramp-like pain in side.
Signs	Loss of the ability to participate; deep breathing.
Special Tests	Not applicable
Referral/ Diagnostic Procedure	Refer to a physician if symptoms/signs persist.
Classification of Injury	Not applicable

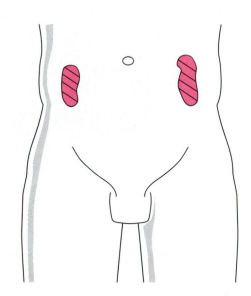

Areas of pain for stitch-in-side condition.

Medical Term	**Peptic ulcer**
Common Term	Same as above
Mechanisms	Excessive production of acid or pepsin; stress.
Symptoms	Vary with the location of the ulcer, such as the stomach or duodenal bulb and the age of the individual. The pain is described as burning, aching, or soreness; it is relieved with antacid medication, food, or milk.
Signs	The pain is located in a well–defined area of epigastric area (region over the pit of the stomach).
Special Tests	Not applicable
Referral/ Diagnostic Procedure	Refer to a physician.
Classification of Injury	Not applicable

HIP INJURIES AND CONDITIONS

Chapter 13

Medical Term	**Iliopectineal bursitis**
Common Term	Same as above
Mechanisms	Overuse as in excessive running; muscle imbalance.
Symptoms	Pain over the anterior aspect of the hip; loss of function; tenderness.
Signs	Pain on flexion, abduction, and external rotation; loss of function; decreased strength; point tenderness; inflammation.
Special Tests	Not applicable
Referral/ Diagnostic Procedure	Refer to an orthopedic surgeon if symptoms/signs persist.
Classification of Injury	Not applicable

Medical Term	**Trochanteric bursitis**
Common Term	Bursitis of the hip
Mechanisms	Trauma to the hip; chronic irritation as in running.
Symptoms	Pain at the hip joint; pain when balancing on the affected leg; loss of hip function; tenderness. The athlete may complain of a "snapping hip."
Signs	Swelling; tenderness; loss of hip function; possible crepitus feeling on palpation; possible increase in the Q-angle in the female athlete; inflammation.
Special Tests	Measure the Q-angle.
Referral/ Diagnostic Procedure	Refer to an orthopedic surgeon if symptoms/signs persist.
Classification of Injury	Not applicable

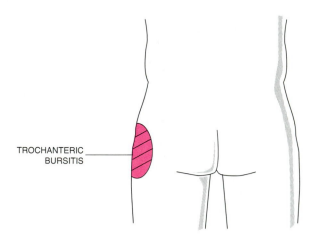

Area of pain for trochanteric bursitis.

Medical Term	**Iliac crest contusion**
Common Term	Hip pointer
Mechanisms	Direct trauma to the iliac crest.
Symptoms	Pain; loss of function; transitory paralysis of hip flexion; tenderness over the crest of the ilium.
Signs	Point tenderness; ecchymosis; hematoma formation; pain on rotation of the trunk; inflammation; loss of hip flexion, muscle spasm.
Special Tests	Assessment of range of motion and strength of hip flexion.
Referral/ Diagnostic Procedure	Refer to an orthopedic surgeon if symptoms/signs persist.
Classification of Injury	First-, second-, and third-degree. See Chapter 1 for classification of contusion injury.

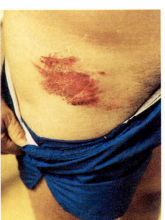 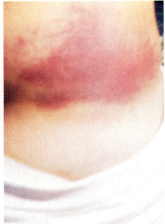 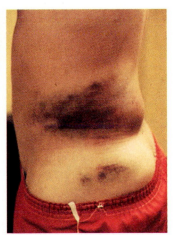

Swelling and ecchymosis from direct trauma to the crest of the ilium, also called a hip pointer.

Medical Term	**Buttocks contusion**
Common Term	Bruised buttocks
Mechanisms	Direct trauma.
Symptoms	Pain; loss of function of hip flexion and extension; transitory paralysis of hip movement; tenderness.
Signs	Point tenderness; possible ecchymosis; hematoma formation; inflammation. Loss of function is minimal because of the protection of fat padding in the area.
Special Tests	Not applicable
Referral/ Diagnostic Procedure	Not applicable
Classification of Injury	First-, second-, and third-degree. See Chapter 1 for classification of contusion injury.

Medical Term	Coccyx contusion
Common Term	Bruised tailbone
Mechanisms	Direct trauma to coccyx from landing on the coccyx in a fall.
Symptoms	Pain when sitting; tenderness over the coccyx.
Signs	Point tenderness over the coccyx; loss of function; ecchymosis; hematoma formation; inflammation; poor walking mechanics; swelling.
Special Tests	Not applicable
Referral/ Diagnostic Procedure	Refer to an orthopedic surgeon. X–ray.
Classification of Injury	First-, second-, and third-degree. See Chapter 1 for classification of contusion injury.

Medical Term	**Coccyx fracture**
Common Term	Broken tailbone
Mechanisms	Direct force to the area of the coccyx, such as an athlete landing in a sitting position on a hard surface.
Symptoms	Unable to sit down without pain; pain to the touch.
Signs	Pain localized above center of buttocks; possible swelling; if pain lasts longer than 72 hours refer to physician for evaluation.
Special Tests	Not applicable
Referral/ Diagnostic Procedure	Refer to a physician for consultation and x–ray.
Classification of Injury	Not applicable

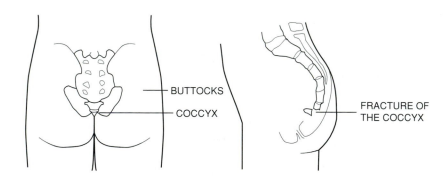

Drawing depicting the location of possible fracture of coccyx.

Medical Term	**Pelvis avulsion fracture**
Common Term	Same as above
Mechanisms	Acute trauma associated with possible severe muscle strain. The site can be at the ischial tuberosity at the hamstring attachment, the anterior superior iliac crest at the attachment of the quadriceps, or the sartorius attachment site.
Symptoms	Sudden pain; loss of function; direct and indirect tenderness.
Signs	Loss of function; direct tenderness; indirect tenderness; swelling; delayed ecchymosis.
Special Tests	Not applicable
Referral/ Diagnostic Procedure	Refer to an orthopedic surgeon. X–ray
Classification of Injury	Not applicable

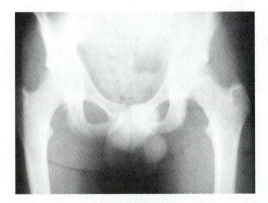

Avulsion fracture of the hamstring attachment.

Medical Term	Pelvis fracture
Common Term	Same as above
Mechanisms	Direct trauma; may be a crushing-type force.
Symptoms	Sudden pain; loss of function; direct and indirect tenderness.
Signs	Loss of function; possible deformity; rapid swelling; direct tenderness; indirect tenderness; possible crepitus; possible false motion; delayed ecchymosis.
Special Tests	Not applicable
Referral/ Diagnostic Procedure	Refer to an orthopedic surgeon. X–ray.
Classification of Injury	Not applicable

A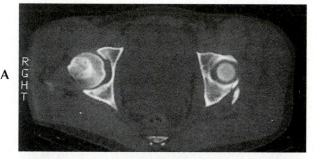

B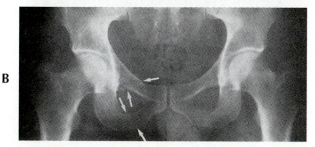

A, CT scan of a posterior fracture of acetabulum of athlete's left hip following a luxation of the hip joint. **B**, Pelvis x-ray of nondisplaced fractures of the pubic rami *(arrows)*.

Medical Term	**Pelvis stress fracture**
Common Term	Same as above
Mechanisms	Overuse; repetitive running.
Symptoms	Point tenderness over the inferior pubic ramus; loss of strength; loss of function; pain in the groin and thigh with exercise that subsides with rest.
Signs	Pain in the groin and referred pain down the thigh; limping; loss of function, inability to stand on the injured leg.
Special Tests	Not applicable
Referral/ Diagnostic Procedure	Refer to an orthopedic surgeon. X–ray, MRI, bone scan.
Classification of Injury	Not applicable

Medical Term	**Legg–Calver–Perthes disease**
Common Term	Coxa plana
Mechanisms	Avascular necrosis of the proximal femoral epiphysis causing a the articular cartilage to become necrotic and flattened; it occurs slowly over a number of months in children 3 to 12 years of age, and it is more common in boys.
Symptoms	Pain in groin sometimes referred to the abdomen and/or knee; loss of normal hip function.
Signs	Walking with a painless limp; loss of range of motion; hip flexion contracture.
Special Tests	Not applicable
Referral/ Diagnostic Procedure	Refer to an orthopedic surgeon. X–ray.
Classification of Injury	Not applicable

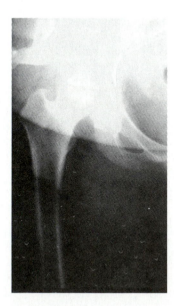

Legg-Calver-Perthes disease demonstrating a small, irregular capital femoral epiphysis.

Medical Term	**Hip luxation**
Common Term	Dislocated hip
Mechanisms	Indirect trauma to the hip joint occuring with a firmly planted foot and an internal rotation force to the femur; the hip is usually flexed and the knee is usually bent. Posterior luxation is most common.
Symptoms	Sudden pain; loss of function.
Signs	Loss of function; point tenderness; marked deformity of the injured leg, which is fixed in hip flexion with an adducted and internally rotated thigh, and the foot of the affected leg resting on the opposite lower leg. The greater trochanter is easily palpated.
Special Tests	Assessment for sciatic nerve involvement. (Refer to lower back chapter for neurologic assessment)
Referral/ Diagnostic Procedure	Refer to an orthopedic surgeon. X–ray for possible fracture.
Classification of Injury	Not applicable

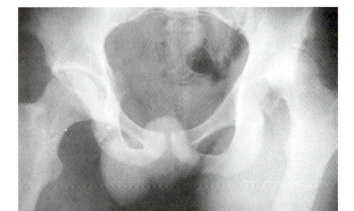

Hip luxation (right side of picture).

Medical Term	Osteitis pubis
Common Term	Inflammed pubic bone
Mechanisms	Overuse and chronic irritation by muscle stress.
Symptoms	Pain in the groin area and symphysis; loss of function; tenderness.
Signs	Pain on palpation of the pubic tubercle; loss of function; direct tenderness; pain on sit-ups, running, and squats; spasm in adductor muscles. The athlete may develop a waddling gait.
Special Tests	Not applicable
Referral/ Diagnostic Procedure	Refer to an orthopedic surgeon. X–ray.
Classification of Injury	Not applicable

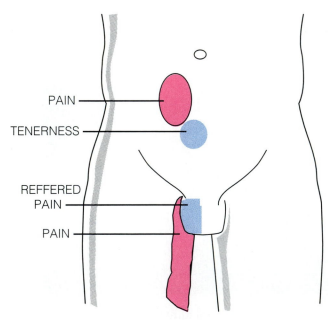

Depiction of area of pain in osteitis pubis.

Medical Term	**Piriformis syndrome**
Common Term	Same as above
Mechanisms	Spasm of the piriformis muscle due to overuse.
Symptoms	Tenderness in the area of the piriformis muscle; pain in the buttocks; loss of normal hip function.
Signs	Sciatic–like symptoms of radiation pain down the leg over dermatome distribution; loss of normal hip function; point tenderness over the piriformis muscle.
Special Tests	Assessment of range of motion and strength test; refer to lower back (Chapter 11) for neurologic assessment.
Referral/ Diagnostic Procedure	Refer to an orthopedic surgeon if symptoms/signs persist.
Classification of Injury	Not applicable

Medical Term	**Capital femoral epiphyseal plate injury**
Common Term	Growth plate injury
Mechanisms	Direct trauma to the hip; indirect trauma as in a twisting motion; could develop over a period of months, and is common in boys between the ages of 10 and 17 who are tall and thin.
Symptoms	Sudden pain; loss of normal hip function.
Signs	Pain on active and passive hip and knee range of motion; loss of normal hip function; limited hip abduction, flexion, and medial rotation; walking with a limp; possible deformity; possible crepitus.
Special Tests	Not applicable
Referral/ Diagnostic Procedure	Refer to an orthopedic surgeon. X–ray.
Classification of Injury	See Chapter 1 for classification of epiphyseal plate injury.

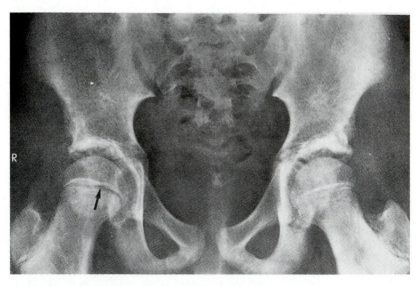

AP view of the pelvis indicating a widened physis of the right femoral head compared to the left *(arrow)*.

Medical Term	Hip sprain
Common Term	Same as above
Mechanisms	Direct trauma from a blow to the hip; overuse as in running or jumping; stretching of the ligamentous structures of the hip joint due to an indirect force applied to the hip joint as with a planted foot and torsion of the leg.
Symptoms	Pain on active movement; pain on passive stress of the ligament; loss of normal hip function; tenderness.
Signs	Point tenderness over the hip joint; swelling; hemorrhage; possible deformity with third-degree injury; ecchymosis; inflammation; walking with a limp; inability to circumduct the hip.
Special Tests	Assessment of range of motion and ligamentous stability test.
Referral/ Diagnostic Procedure	Refer to an orthopedic surgeon if symptoms/signs persist.
Classification of Injury	First-, second-, and third-degree. See Chapter 1 for classification of sprain injury.

Medical Term	Hip strain
Common Term	Same as above
Mechanisms	Trauma to the musculotendinous unit due to excessive contraction or stretching; predisposing muscle fatigue.
Symptoms	Pain on active movement of the hip; pain on passive stretch of the hip; loss of normal hip function; possible snapping sound heard when the injury occurs; muscle fatigue before the injury; tenderness.
Signs	Muscle spasm; loss of range of motion; swelling; ecchymosis; loss of strength; hematoma formation; possible defect in musculotendinous unit in third-degree injury; point tenderness.
Special Tests	Assessment of range of motion and strength test; Trendelenburg test; Thomas test; Kendall test.
Referral/ Diagnostic Procedure	Refer to an orthopedic surgeon if symptoms/signs persist.
Classification of Injury	First-, second-, and third-degree. See Chapter 1 for classification of strain injury.

Medical Term	**Synovitis of the hip**
Common Term	Same as above
Mechanisms	Direct trauma; torsion.
Symptoms	Pain in the hip; loss of function; pain down the lateral side of the leg.
Signs	Loss of function; swelling; loss of strength.
Special Tests	Not applicable
Referral/ Diagnostic Procedure	Refer to an orthopedic surgeon if symptoms/signs persist.
Classification of Injury	Not applicable

Medical Term	**Hip tendinitis**
Common Term	Same as above
Mechanisms	Overuse; poor mechanics in activity; degenerative changes.
Symptoms	Pain on active movement of the hip; pain on passive stretch of the hip; loss of normal hip function; overuse activity such as running; tenderness.
Signs	Swelling; loss of normal hip function; possible crepitus; inflammation; point tenderness.
Special Tests	Assessment of range of motion and strength test.
Referral/ Diagnostic Procedure	Refer to an orthopedic surgeon if symptoms/signs persist.
Classification of Injury	Not applicable

■ TESTS FOR EVALUATION OF INJURIES TO THE HIP ■

(Perform all tests bilaterally)

■ GENERAL ASSESSMENT TEST FOR RANGE OF MOTION AND STRENGTH FOR A STRAIN, TENDINITIS, AND TENOSYNOVITIS

Active Movement

The athlete moves the body part through the range of motion actively, trying to reproduce the pain.

Passive Stretch

The athletic trainer performs a passive stretch of the involved muscle or tendon.

Resistive Movement

The athlete moves the body part through the range of motion while the athletic trainer applies resistance.

■ GENERAL ASSESSMENT TEST FOR RANGE OF MOTION AND LIGAMENTOUS STABILITY FOR A SPRAIN

Active Movement

The athlete moves the joint through the range of motion actively. The athletic trainer should be looking for any limitations in the range of motion.

Passive Movement

If the athlete cannot move the joint through the range of motion actively, then passive range of motion should be done to determine whether the range of motion is blocked due to the athlete's pain or because some object is blocking the joint.

Resistive Movement

The athlete moves the joint through the range of motion while the athletic trainer applies resistance.

Passive Stress

The athletic trainer applies stress to the joint to test the integrity of the ligamentous structures of the joint.

■ TEST FOR THE STRENGTH OF THE GLUTEUS MEDIUS MUSCLE

Trendelenburg Test

The athletic trainer should stand behind the athlete and observe the posterior iliac spine. The athletic trainer should ask the athlete to lift one leg. Standing erect, the gluteus medius on the supporting leg should contract when the opposite foot leaves the ground and elevates the pelvis on the unsupported side.

■ TEST FOR HIP FLEXION CONTRACTURE

Kendall Test

Lie the athlete supine on the table with the uninvolved knee flexed to the chest and the back flat. Place the other knee over the end of the table. The thigh of the involved leg should touch the table with the knee flexed at about 70°. The test is positive if the thigh does not lie flat on the table.

Thomas Test

Lie the athlete supine on the table, arms crossed over the chest and the legs fully extended. The athletic trainer places one hand under the lumbar spine and instructs the athlete to bring the knee of one leg to the chest. The other leg should remain flat on the table; if it does not; there is a hip contracture.

THIGH INJURIES AND CONDITIONS

Chapter 14

Medical Term	**Ilium apophysitis**
Common Term	Inflammation of apophysis
Mechanisms	Overuse as in long-distance running; apophysitis can occur at the ischial tuberosity, the anterior inferior iliac spine, or the anterior superior iliac spine. It can lead to avulsion fracture.
Symptoms	Pain at site of apophysis; loss of normal hip function.
Signs	Loss of strength; loss of normal hip function; point tenderness of the ischial tuberosity, anterior inferior iliac spine or anterior superior iliac spine.
Special Tests	Not applicable
Referral/ Diagnostic Procedure	Refer to an orthopedic surgeon. X–ray.
Classification of Injury	Not applicable

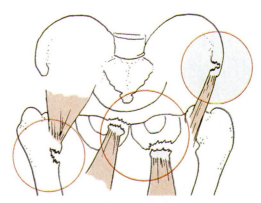

Sites of apophysitis of the pelvis.

Medical Term	**Thigh contusion**
Common Term	Charley horse
Mechanisms	Direct trauma.
Symptoms	Pain in anterior thigh; loss of function of the quadriceps; transitory paralysis of the quadriceps; tenderness.
Signs	Point tenderness; ecchymosis; hematoma formation; inflammation; loss of quadricep function; loss of strength; swelling may appear in knee as fluid; third-degree can lead to myositis ossificans.
Special Tests	Assessment of range of motion and strength test.
Referral/ Diagnostic Procedure	Refer to an orthopedic surgeon if symptoms/signs persist. X–ray.
Classification of Injury	First-, second-, and third-degree. See Chapter 1 for classification of contusion injury.

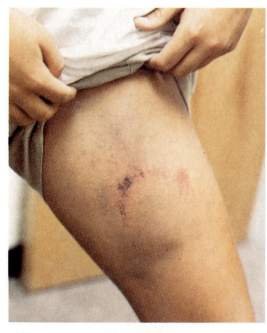

Ecchymosis due to contusion of the thigh.

Medical Term	**Proximal femur epiphyseal plate injury**
Common Term	Same as above
Mechanisms	Direct trauma causing a shearing force. This injury occurs in individuals 10 to 16 years of age.
Symptoms	Pain; loss of normal hip function; pain on weight bearing.
Signs	Loss of function; rapid swelling; possible deformity; direct tenderness; indirect tenderness; possible bony deviations; possible crepitus; possible false joint motion; delayed ecchymosis.
Special Tests	Not applicable
Referral/ Diagnostic Procedure	Refer to an orthopedic surgeon. X–ray.
Classification of Injury	See Chapter 1 for classification of epiphyseal plate injury.

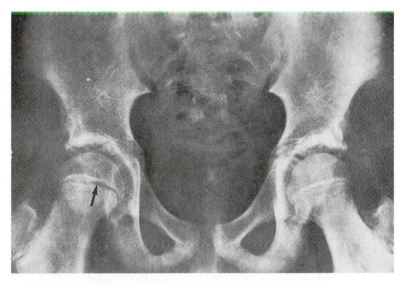

Epiphyseal plate fracture of the proximal femur.

Medical Term	Quadriceps attachment avulsion fracture
Common Term	Fracture
Mechanisms	Indirect trauma as in a violent, sudden, explosive movement with contraction of the quadriceps or from an over stretch of the quadriceps.
Symptoms	Pain at the site of the avulsion; loss of normal hip flexion and knee extension; loss of strength; tenderness. This type of injury is more common in young athletes due to the attachment of the quadriceps at the apophysitis of the hip.
Signs	Point tenderness; loss of strength; loss of normal hip flexion and knee extension; defect may be felt at the point of the quadriceps attachment to the ilium.
Special Tests	Not applicable
Referral/ Diagnostic Procedure	Refer to an orthopedic surgeon. X–ray.
Classification of Injury	Not applicable

Medical Term	Femur fracture
Common Term	Broken leg
Mechanisms	Direct trauma from a blow applied to the femur, such as in tackling in football; indirect force, such as in landing on an extended leg or torsion.
Symptoms	Sudden severe pain; loss of function; direct and indirect tenderness.
Signs	Loss of function; possible deformity; rapid swelling; possible shock; direct tenderness; indirect tenderness; possible bony deviation; possible crepitus; possible false joint motion; possible shortened leg; thigh outwardly rotated; delayed ecchymosis.
Special Tests	Check pulse at the posterior tibial artery.
Referral/ Diagnostic Procedure	Refer to an orthopedic surgeon. X–ray.
Classification of Injury	Not applicable

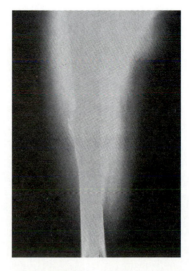

Fractured femur.

Medical Term	**Femur stress fracture / femoral neck**
Common Term	Same as above
Mechanisms	Overuse as in repetitive activity such as long-distance running.
Symptoms	Pain at the femoral neck; loss of normal function. Pain subsides with rest.
Signs	Tenderness at the femoral neck; nonspecific pain that may be referred to the groin or knee; noticeable limp that is progressive; loss of normal function; persistent pain.
Special Tests	Not applicable
Referral/ Diagnostic Procedure	Refer to an orthopedic surgeon. X–ray; bone scan.
Classification of Injury	Not applicable

Medical Term	**Iliopsoas bursitis**
Common Term	Bursitis
Mechanisms	Overuse; excessive running.
Symptoms	Pain over the anterior portion of the hip; loss of normal hip flexion, abduction and external rotation; tenderness.
Signs	Pain on flexion, abduction, and external rotation of the hip; decrease in strength; tenderness; inflammation.
Special Tests	Not applicable
Referral/ Diagnostic Procedure	Refer to an orthopedic surgeon if symptoms/signs persist.
Classification of Injury	Not applicable

Medical Term   Myositis ossificans

Common Term   Calcium deposit

Mechanisms   Direct trauma to the muscle causing bleeding; over aggressive quadriceps mobilization during the early stages of rehabilitation after a quadricecps contusion; repeated instances of reinjury.

Symptoms   Pain; loss of knee flexion or extension.

Signs   Mass felt within the quadriceps muscle or hamstring, usually three to four weeks post injury; tenderness; loss of function of knee flexion or extension.

Special Tests   Assessment of range of motion and strength test.

Referral/   Refer to an orthopedic surgeon. X–ray four weeks post
Diagnostic   injury.
Procedure

Classification   See Chapter 1 for classification of third degree contusion.
of Injury

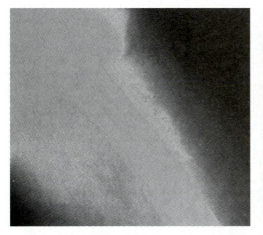 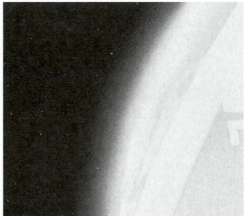

Myositis ossificans in the quadriceps muscle.

Medical Term	**Snapping hip**
Common Term	Hurdler or dance hip
Mechanisms	Overuse movements that predisposes an imbalance of the muscles of the hip; lateral rotation and flexion of the hip joint as in a dance movement; related to structural narrow biiliac width.
Symptoms	Athlete complains of snapping sensation at the hip; pain in the hip.
Signs	Inflammation; greater than normal range of motion in hip abduction; restricted range of motion in lateral rotation.
Special Tests	Not applicable
Referral/ Diagnostic Procedure	Refer to an orthopedic surgeon.
Classification of Injury	Not applicable

Medical Term	Hamstring strain
Common Term	Pulled hamstring
Mechanisms	Trauma to the hamstring musculotendinous unit resulting from excessive forcible contraction or stretching; predisposing muscle fatigue; poor muscle coordination.
Symptoms	Pain that increases with active and resistive movement; pain on passive stretch; loss of knee flexion; possible snapping sound heard when the injury occurs; muscle fatigue before injury; tenderness.
Signs	Muscle spasm; swelling; ecchymosis; point tenderness; loss of knee flexion; loss of strength; hematoma formation and possible defect in the musculotendinous unit in third degree injury; inflammation; poor flexibility in hamstrings.
Special Tests	Assessment of range of motion and strength test.
Referral/ Diagnostic Procedure	Refer to an orthopedic surgeon is symptoms/signs persist.
Classification of Injury	First-, second-, and third-degree. See Chapter 1 for classification of strain injury.

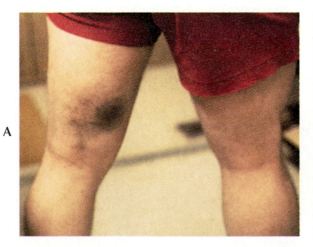
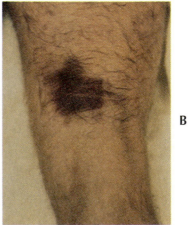

A and **B**, Swelling and ecchymosis following first-degree hamstring strain.

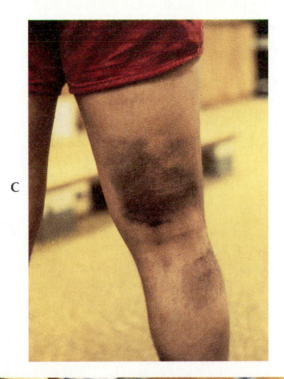

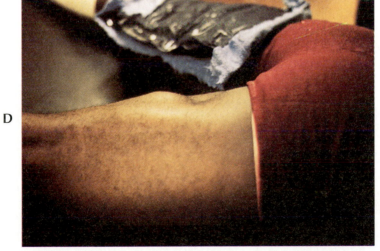

C, Swelling and ecchymosis following second-degree hamstring strain. **D,** Rupture of hamstring muscle (third-degree strain).

Medical Term	Quadriceps strain
Common Term	Pulled thigh muscle
Mechanisms	Indirect trauma to the quadriceps musculotendinous unit resulting from excessive contraction or stretching; predisposing muscle fatigue.
Symptoms	Pain increased with active and resistive movement; pain on passive stretch; loss of knee extension; possible snapping sound heard when the injury occurs; muscle fatigue before the injury occurs; tenderness.
Signs	Muscle spasms; swelling; possible ecchymosis; point tenderness; loss of knee extension; loss of strength; hematoma formation and defect in the musculotendinous unit with third-degree injury; inflammation.
Special Tests	Assessment of range of motion and strength test.
Referral/ Diagnostic Procedure	Refer to an orthopedic surgeon if symptoms/signs persist.
Classification of Injury	First-, second-, and third-degree. See Chapter 1 for classification of strain injury.

Medical Term	Tendinitis
Common Term	Same as above
Mechanisms	Overuse; poor mechanics in running; degenerative changes.
Symptoms	Pain on active and resistive movements; pain on passive stretch; loss of function; overuse activity.
Signs	Swelling; loss of function; possible crepitus; possible calcium formation; inflammation.
Special Tests	Assessment of range of motion and strength test.
Referral/ Diagnostic Procedure	Refer to an orthopedic surgeon if symptoms/signs persist.
Classification of Injury	Not applicable

■ TESTS FOR EVALUATION OF INJURIES TO THE ■ PELVIC/THIGH AREA

(All tests should be performed bilaterally)

■ GENERAL ASSESSMENT FOR RANGE OF MOTION AND STRENGTH FOR STRAIN, TENDINITIS, AND TENOSYNOVITIS

Active Movement

The athlete moves the body part through the range of motion actively, trying to reproduce the pain.

Passive Stretch

The athletic trainer performs a passive stretch of the involved muscle or tendon.

Resistive Movement

The athlete moves the body part through the range of motion while the athletic trainer applies resistance.

■ GENERAL ASSESSMENT TEST FOR RANGE OF MOTION AND LIGAMENTOUS STABILITY FOR A SPRAIN

Active Movement

The athlete moves the joint through the range of motion actively. The athletic trainer should be looking for any limitations in the range of motion.

Passive Movement

If the athlete cannot move the joint through the range of motion actively, then passive range of motion should be done to determine whether the range of motion is blocked due to the athlete's pain or because some object is blocking the joint.

Resistive Movement

The athlete moves the joint through the range of motion, while the athletic trainer applies resistance.

Passive Stress

The athletic trainer applies stress to the joint to test the integrity of the ligamentous structures of the joint.

KNEE INJURIES AND CONDITIONS

Chapter 15

Suprapatellar Bursitis

Infrapatella Bursitis

Pes Anserine Bursitis

Chondral/Osteochondral Fracture

Chondromalacia Patella

Tibiofemoral Luxation

Acute Patella Luxation

Recurrent Patella Luxation

Distal Femur Epiphyseal Plate
  Injury/Fracture

Lateral Meniscal Tear

Iliotibial Band Friction Syndrome

Patella Fracture

Hoffa's Disease

Popliteal Cyst

Peroneal Nerve Contusion

Patellar Tendon Rupture

Osgood–Schlatter Condition

Sinding–Larsen–Johansson Condition

Osteochondritis Dissecans

Knee Synovitis

Sprain/Straight Posterior Instability

Sprain/Straight Varus Instability

Sprain/Straight Anterior Instability

Sprain/Valgus Instability

Sprain/Anteromedial Rotary
  Instability

Sprain/Anterolateral Rotary
  Instability

Sprain/Posterolateral Instability

Plica Irritation

Knee Contusion

Medial Meniscal Tear

Pes Anserine Tendinitis

Popliteus Tendinitis

Patella Tendinitis

Medical Term	**Suprapatellar bursitis**
Common Term	Housemaid's knee; carpet layer's knee
Mechanisms	Overuse; direct trauma as in continued kneeling in wrestling.
Symptoms	Pain; loss of normal knee flexion and extension; tenderness.
Signs	Redness; swelling; loss of normal knee flexion and extension; point tenderness over the suprapatellar bursa; inflammation; possible calcium formation in chronic cases.
Special Tests	Assessment of range of motion and strength.
Referral/ Diagnostic Procedure	Refer to an orthopedic surgeon.
Classification of Injury	Not applicable

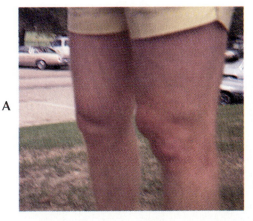 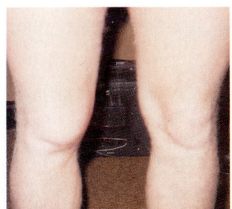

A and B, Swelling above the patella due to suprapatellar bursitis.

Medical Term	**Infrapatellar bursitis**
Common Term	Jumper's knee
Mechanisms	Overuse as in continuous jumping; direct trauma as in a contusion to the area.
Symptoms	Pain below the patella; loss of knee extension and flexion; tenderness.
Signs	Redness; swelling; loss of knee extension and flexion; point tenderness over the infrapatellar bursa; inflammation; possible calcium formation in chronic cases.
Special Tests	Assessment of range of motion and strength.
Referral/ Diagnostic Procedure	Refer to an orthopedic surgeon.
Classification of Injury	Not applicable

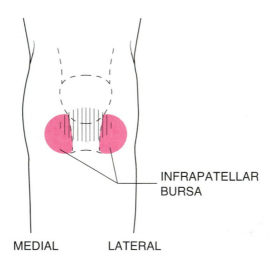

Lines show typical area of pain for infrapatellar bursitis.

Medical Term	**Pes anserine bursitis**
Common Term	Pretibial bursitis
Mechanisms	Overuse as in long distance running; direct trauma such as a blow to the medial side of the knee.
Symptoms	Pain; loss of normal knee flexion, extension, and internal rotation; tenderness.
Signs	Redness; swelling; loss of normal knee flexion, extension, and internal rotation; point tenderness over the pes anserine bursa on the medial tibial plateau; inflammation.
Special Tests	Assessment of range of motion and strength.
Referral/ Diagnostic Procedure	Refer to an orthopedic surgeon.
Classification of Injury	Not applicable

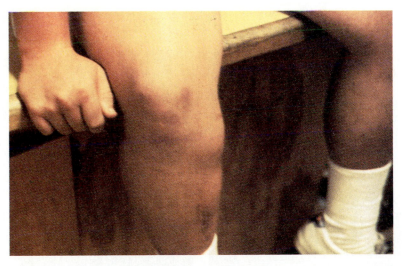

Swelling over the pes anserine bursae, indicating pes anserine bursitis.

Medical Term	Chondral/osteochondral fracture
Common Term	Same as above
Mechanisms	Indirect compressive or shearing forces that are associated with knee torsion.
Symptoms	Sudden pain in the knee joint; loss of normal knee movement; locking; pain on flexion and extension; pain on manual pressure against the femoral condyles; snapping; buckling.
Signs	Loss of normal knee movement; effusion of the knee joint; joint line tenderness; inability to fully extend the knee; possible bony deviations; possible crepitus; delayed ecchymosis.
Special Tests	Not applicable
Referral/ Diagnostic Procedure	Refer to an orthopedic surgeon. X–ray, MRI.
Classification of Injury	Not applicable

A 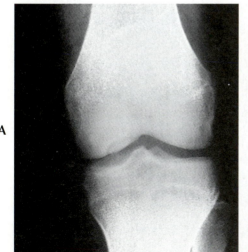 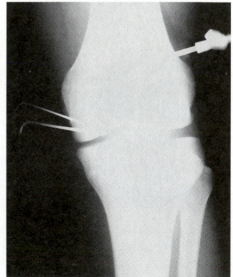 B

A, Osteochondral fracture fragment of the femoral condyle. **B**, Osteochondral fracture fragment repair with pinning.

Medical Term	Chondromalacia patella
Common Term	Same as above
Mechanisms	Repeated direct trauma to the patella as in recurrent subluxation; predisposing factors may include malalignment of extensor mechanism of the knee, leg length, or abnormal pronation of the ankle.
Symptoms	Pain under the patella upon flexion and extension of the knee; tenderness along the medial border and articular surface of the patella; slight stiffness of the knee joint; pain when walking up and down stairs.
Signs	Temporary loss of function; instability; swelling; subpatellar crepitation on active movement; atrophy of the quadriceps; predisposing Q-angle greater than 18° to 20°; tenderness along the medial border and articular surface of the patella.
Special Tests	Patella grind test; patella compression test; measure Q-angle.
Referral/ Diagnostic Procedure	Refer to an orthopedic surgeon. X–ray, MRI.
Classification of Injury	Not applicable

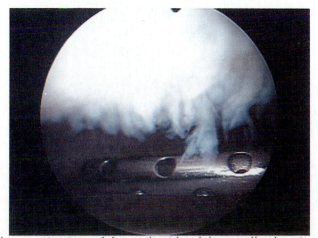

Arthroscopic view of the underside of the patella showing degenerative changes (ruffening) indicating chondromalacia.

Medical Term   Tibiofemoral luxation

Common Term   Dislocated knee

Mechanisms   Direct force to the front of the leg near the knee; excessive forcible hyperextension; lateral leverage forces.

Symptoms   Pain; loss of normal knee function; tenderness.

Signs   Marked deformity; loss of normal knee function; swelling; point tenderness; abnormal laxity in the knee; delayed ecchymosis.

Special Tests   Check dorsal pedal and posterior tibial pulses; check for normal neurologic sensation.

Referral/ Diagnostic Procedure   Refer to an orthopedic surgeon.

Classification of Injury   Not applicable

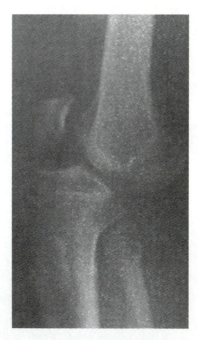

Luxation of the tibiofemoral joint.

Medical Term	**Acute patella luxation**
Common Term	Dislocated kneecap
Mechanisms	Violent force against the medial aspect to the patella from a forcible rotation of the femur on a fixed tibia; lateral rotation of the tibia on a fixed femur; a direct fall in extension, contraction of the quadriceps.
Symptoms	Pain; loss of function; snapping or popping sound heard when the injury occurs; the athlete complains of the knee "giving away."
Signs	Marked deformity with displaced patella; abducted tibia; tenderness on the medial aspect to the patella; swelling; delayed ecchymosis. The patella may reduce spontaneously if the knee is straightened.
Special Tests	Apprehension test.
Referral/ Diagnostic Procedure	Refer to an orthopedic surgeon. X–ray.
Classification of Injury	Not applicable

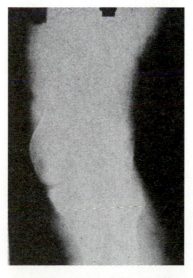

Lateral luxation of the patella
(right side of picture).

Medical Term	Recurrent patella luxation
Common Term	Dislocated kneecap
Mechanisms	Direct trauma as in a blow to the medial or lateral side of the patella; predisposing factors include bony arrangement, Q-angle greater than 18° to 20°, high riding patella, shallow intercondyle groove, weak vastus medialis.
Symptoms	Pain at the patella; loss of normal knee function; popping or snapping sound heard when the injury occurs; tenderness.
Signs	Displacement of the patella, usually lateral; atrophy of the vastus medialis; laxity in the medial joint capsule; loss of normal knee function; swelling; inflammation; point tenderness over the medial aspect of the patella.
Special Tests	Apprehension test, measure Q-angle.
Referral/ Diagnostic Procedure	Refer to an orthopedic surgeon. X–ray.
Classification of Injury	Not applicable

Medical Term	**Distal femur epiphyseal plate injury/fracture**
Common Term	Same as above
Mechanisms	Direct trauma as in a blow to the knee with a valgus force; indirect trauma as in a shearing force; occurs in individuals 10 to 16 years of age.
Symptoms	Pain; loss of function; pain on weight bearing; tenderness 3 or 4 inches (7.5 to 10 cm) above joint line.
Signs	Loss of function; rapid swelling; possible deformity; direct tenderness; indirect tenderness; possible bony deviations; possible crepitus; possible false motion 3 to 4 inches above the joint line; delayed ecchymosis; possible leg length discrepancy.
Special Tests	Not applicable
Referral/ Diagnostic Procedure	Refer to an orthopedic surgeon. X–ray.
Classification of Injury	See Chapter 1 for classification of epiphyseal plate injury.

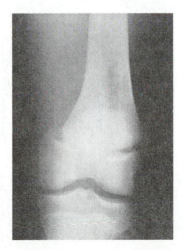

X-ray of an epiphyseal plate fracture of the distal femur in a 14-year-old football athlete.

Medical Term	**Lateral meniscal tear**
Common Term	Torn cartilage
Mechanisms	Indirect forces such as internal rotation of a planted foot and lower leg; hyperextension of the knee; hyperflexion of the knee; cutting motion; prolonged overuse.
Symptoms	Pain; periodic locking; sensation of the knee "giving way"; possible clicking sensation when walking up or down stairs; pain when squatting.
Signs	Lateral joint pain; swelling; weakened or atrophied quadriceps muscle; possible locking.
Special Tests	McMurry's test; Apley's compression test; modified Apley's compression test; bounce home test.
Referral/ Diagnostic Procedure	Not applicable
Classification of Injury	Not applicable

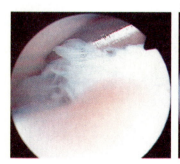 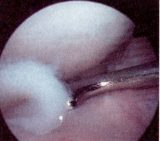 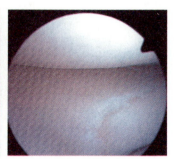

A, Arthroscopic view of a torn lateral meniscus. "String" appearance of the edge of the meniscus indicates the tear. **B,** Arthroscopic view of a lateral meniscus tear indicated by the inner edge of the meniscus being pulled away from its normal attachment to the body of the lateral meniscus. **C,** Arthroscopic view of the inner edge of the lateral meniscus after repair.

Medical Term	**Iliotibial band friction syndrome**
Common Term	Same as above
Mechanisms	Overuse as in long-distance running causing an irritation from friction of the iliotibial band over the lateral femoral epicondyle.
Symptoms	Discomfort, ranging from a dull ache to sharp pain on the lateral aspect of the knee; pain that increases with running on uneven terrain; pain that increases with knee flexion and extension while weight bearing.
Signs	Tenderness over the lateral femoral epicondyle on palpation; clicking sensation on palpation over the lateral femoral epicondyle with weight bearing at 30° of knee flexion.
Special Tests	Ober's test.
Referral/ Diagnostic Procedure	Palpate the lateral femoral epicondyle with weight bearing at 30° of flexion.
Classification of Injury	Not applicable

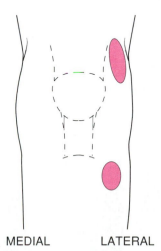

MEDIAL   LATERAL

Drawing showing areas of pain for iliotibial band tendinitis.

Medical Term	Patella fracture
Common Term	Broken kneecap
Mechanisms	Direct trauma to the patella as in a fall; indirect trauma as in a severe pull of the patella tendon. This fracture occurs against the femur with the knee semiflexed.
Symptoms	Sudden pain; loss of normal knee flexion and extension; direct and indirect tenderness of the patella.
Signs	Loss of normal knee flexion and extension; possible deformity; rapid swelling; direct tenderness; indirect tenderness; possible bony deviation; possible crepitus; possible false joint motion; delayed ecchymosis.
Special Tests	Not applicable
Referral/ Diagnostic Procedure	Refer to an orthopedic surgeon. X–ray.
Classification of Injury	Not applicable

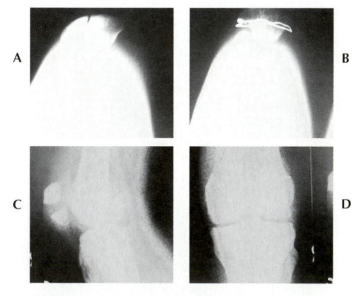

A, Sunrise view of longitudinal fracture of the patella on x-ray. **B**, Repair of patella fracture. **C**, Transverse fracture of the patella. **D**, Repair of transverse fracture of the patella.

Medical Term	**Hoffa's disease**
Common Term	Fat pad contusion
Mechanisms	Direct trauma as in a fall on the knee; indirect trauma from the pad being caught between the femoral condyles and the tibial plateaus on extension or repeated kneeling.
Symptoms	Pain; tenderness medial and lateral to the patella tendon; loss of normal knee function.
Signs	Swelling inferior to the patella; point tenderness medial and lateral to the patella tendon; loss of normal knee function; inflammation.
Special Tests	Not applicable
Referral/ Diagnostic Procedure	Refer to an orthopedic surgeon if symptoms/signs persist.
Classification of Injury	Not applicable

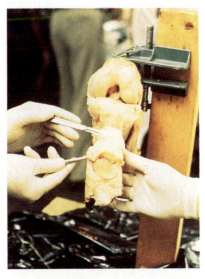

Pointer indicates the infrapatellar
fat pad involved in Hoffa's disease.

Medical Term	**Popliteal cyst**
Common Term	Baker's cyst
Mechanisms	Posterior damage to the medial meniscus; hernia of the semitendinous sheath; deterioration of the posterior capsule. The contents of the bursal sac may discharge into the knee, causing synovitis.
Symptoms	Pain; loss of normal knee function.
Signs	Large soft tissue on the medial side in the popliteal space; periodic swelling.
Special Tests	Not applicable
Referral/ Diagnostic Procedure	Refer to an orthopedic surgeon. MRI.
Classification of Injury	Not applicable

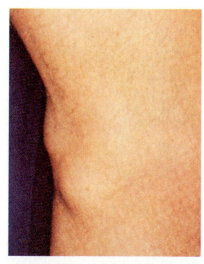

Popliteal cysts (Baker's cyst) as indicated by swelling in the posterior aspect of the knee.

Medical Term	**Peroneal nerve contusion**
Common Term	Same as above
Mechanisms	Direct trauma to the proximal fibula.
Symptoms	Immediate severe local pain; electric shock sensation radiating to anterior and lateral leg and the dorsum of the foot; numbness and tingling; tenderness of the underlying nerve.
Signs	Edema; possible paresthesia with resulting drop foot; possible paralysis; point tenderness over the peroneal nerve.
Special Tests	Assessment of range of motion and strength, especially the ankle dorsiflexors and evertors; neurological assessment of the peroneal nerve.
Referral/ Diagnostic Procedure	Refer to a neurologist. EMG studies.
Classification of Injury	Not applicable

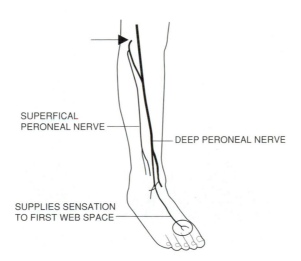

SUPERFICAL PERONEAL NERVE

DEEP PERONEAL NERVE

SUPPLIES SENSATION TO FIRST WEB SPACE

Arrow shows usual point of trauma and circle demonstrates the area of sensation loss.

Medical Term	**Patellar tendon rupture**
Common Term	Same as above
Mechanisms	Indirect force as in landing in an off-balance position causing a violent contraction of the quadriceps.
Symptoms	Sudden, sharp pain; loss of quadriceps function; a snap or pop heard when the injury occurs; tenderness.
Signs	Patella sitting proximal (high-riding patella); point tenderness at the site of the rupture; defect that can be felt in the area of the patella tendon; loss of knee extension.
Special Tests	Assessment of range of motion and strength.
Referral/ Diagnostic Procedure	Refer to an orthopedic surgeon.
Classification of Injury	Not applicable

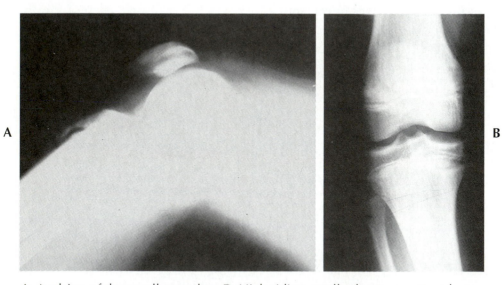

A, Avulsion of the patellar tendon. **B**, High-riding patella due to a ruptured patellar tendon.

Medical Term	Osgood–Schlatter condition
Common Term	Same as above
Mechanisms	Overuse such as repetitive stress on the patella tendon, causing avulsion at the tibial tuberosity. This condition may be related to a growth spurt in athletes in prepubertal stage of development.
Symptoms	Pain on active movement of the quadriceps; point tenderness below the knee at the tibial tuberosity; pain on squatting; pain on resistive movement of the quadriceps.
Signs	Quadriceps atrophy; prominent tibial epiphysis; point tenderness on palpation of the tibial tuberosity; swelling; inflammation.
Special Tests	Not applicable
Referral/ Diagnostic Procedure	Refer to an orthopedic surgeon. X–ray.
Classification of Injury	Not applicable

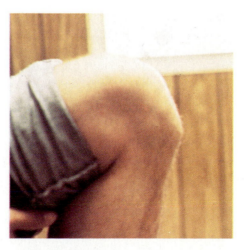

Osgood-Schlatter condition is indicated by the bony prominence at the tibial tuberosity.

Medical Term	Sinding–Larsen–Johansson condition
Common Term	Same as above
Mechanisms	Overuse of the patella tendon.
Symptoms	Pain on kneeling or activity; loss of normal knee function; tenderness at the inferior pole of the patella; pain on active and resistive movement. This condition is most common in youths 10 to 12 years of age.
Signs	Pain at the inferior pole of the patella; swelling; point tenderness; possible bony irregularity at the patella tendon origin.
Special Tests	Assessment of range of motion and strength.
Referral/ Diagnostic Procedure	Refer to an orthopedic surgeon.
Classification of Injury	Not applicable

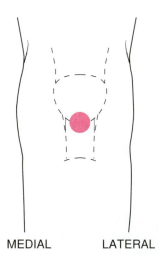

MEDIAL   LATERAL

Area of pain for Sinding-Larsen-Johannson condition.

Medical Term	Osteochondritis dissecans
Common Term	Joint mice
Mechanisms	Unknown; impairment of the blood supply to the affected segment of bone causing a degeneration of the articular cartilage.
Symptoms	Pain after exercise; loss of function; chronic, nonspecific, intermittent locking.
Signs	Chronic, nonspecific swelling; loss of function; muscle atrophy; possible crepitus; transient locking; possible palpation of loose bodies.
Special Tests	Not applicable
Referral/ Diagnostic Procedure	Refer to an orthopedic surgeon. X–ray, MRI.
Classification of Injury	Not applicable

Medical Term	Knee synovitis
Common Term	Water on the knee
Mechanisms	Trauma; contusion; sprain; irritation from floating of cartilage.
Symptoms	Pain after activity; loss of function; tenderness.
Signs	Swelling; loss of function; erythema; tenderness; muscle spasm; patella floating up from condyles due to swelling (ballottable patella).
Special Tests	Ballottable patella test.
Referral/ Diagnostic Procedure	Refer to an orthopedic surgeon.
Classification of Injury	Not applicable

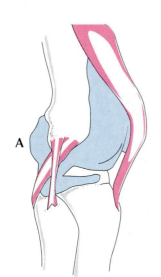 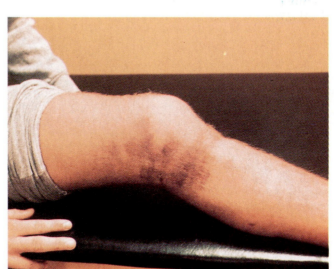

A, Blue area denotes the synovial membrane of the knee. **B**, Swelling and ecchymosis due to synovitis of the knee.

Medical Term	**Sprain/Straight posterior instability**
Common Term	PCL sprain
Mechanisms	Indirect trauma that forces the tibia posterior in relation to the femur as in hyperflexion, hyperextension, abduction/valgus force, causing a stretching of the posterior cruciate ligament or posterior capsule.
Symptoms	Pain on active movement; pain on passive stress; loss of normal knee function; pain on resistive movements; tenderness.
Signs	Swelling; hemorrhage; instability with second- and third-degree injury; loss of normal knee function; inflammation; posterior subluxation of the tibia on the femur.
Special Tests	Posterior drawer stress test; Lachman's test; gravity drawer test.
Referral/ Diagnostic Procedure	Refer to an orthopedic surgeon. MRI.
Classification of Injury	First-, second-, and third-degree. See Chapter 1 for classification of sprain injury.

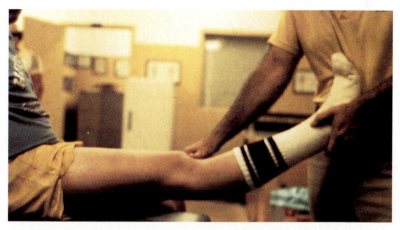

Hyperextension of the knee due to posterior instability.

Medical Term	**Sprain/Straight varus instability**
Common Term	LCL sprain
Mechanisms	Varus force applied to an adducted, internally rotated tibia; rotation, stretching of the fibular collateral ligament due to direct or indirect force applied to the knee joint.
Symptoms	Pain on active movement; pain on passive stress; loss of normal knee function; pain on resistive movement; tenderness.
Signs	Point tenderness over the fibular collateral ligament; swelling; hemorrhage; lateral instability of the knee joint with second and third degree injury; inflammation; loss of normal knee function.
Special Tests	Assessment of range of motion and ligamentous stability with a varus (adduction) stress test.
Referral/ Diagnostic Procedure	Refer to an orthopedic surgeon. MRI.
Classification of Injury	First-, second-, and third-degree. See Chapter 1 for classification of sprain injury.

Medical Term	Sprain/Straight anterior instability
Common Term	ACL sprain
Mechanisms	Indirect force causing internal rotation of the femur with the knee flexed and the foot planted or hyperextension of the knee.
Symptoms	Pain on active movement; pain on passive stress; loss of normal knee function; pain on resistive movement.
Signs	Point tenderness at the attachment of the anterior cruciate ligament on the tibia; swelling; hemorrhage; anterior instability of the knee with second- and third-degree injury; inflammation; loss of normal knee function.
Special Tests	Anterior drawer test; Lachman's test; gravity drawer test, lateral pivot shift test.
Referral/ Diagnostic Procedure	Refer to an orthopedic surgeon. MRI.
Classification of Injury	First-, second-, and third-degree. See Chapter 1 for classification of sprain injury.

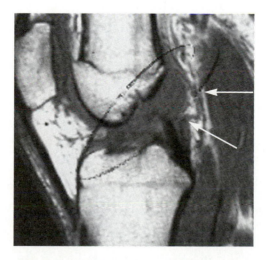

MRI showing disruption of ACL fibers
(arrows).

Medical Term	**Sprain/Valgus instability**
Common Term	MCL sprain
Mechanisms	Indirect trauma to the tibial collateral ligament due to a valgus force applied to the knee joint, with the foot planted and the tibia externally rotated and abducted. Overuse as with the breast stroke in swimming.
Symptoms	Pain on active and resistive movement of the knee joint; pain on passive stress; loss of normal knee function.
Signs	Point tenderness over the tibial collateral ligament; swelling; hemorrhage; ecchymosis; medial knee instability with second- and third-degree injury; inflammation; loss of normal knee function.
Special Tests	Assessment of range of motion and ligamentous stability with the valgus (abduction) stress test at full (0°) extension and with 30° of flexion.
Referral/ Diagnostic Procedure	Refer to an orthopedic surgeon. MRI.
Classification of Injury	First-, second-, and third-degree. See Chapter 1 for classification of sprain injury.

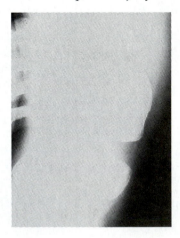

Stress x-ray indicating
medial joint laxity during
valgus stress test.

Medical Term	**Sprain/Anteromedial rotary instability**
Common Term	Same as above
Mechanisms	Indirect lateral trauma to the knee with the tibia in external rotation and the foot firmly planted, stretching the anterior cruciate ligament and medial capsule.
Symptoms	Pain on active movement; pain on passive stress; loss of normal knee function; pain on resistive movement; tenderness.
Signs	Point tenderness over the attachment of the anterior cruciate ligament attachment on the tibia; swelling; hemorrhage; possible deformity with third degree injury; anterior rotary instability with second and third degree injury; inflammation; ecchymosis; loss of normal knee function.
Special Tests	Assessment of range of motion and ligamentous stability to include the slocum external rotation test and valgus (abduction) stress test.
Referral/ Diagnostic Procedure	Refer to an orthopedic surgeon. MRI.
Classification of Injury	First-, second-, and third-degree. See Chapter 1 for classification of sprain injury.

Medical Term	Sprain/Anterolateral rotary instability
Common Term	Same as above
Mechanisms	Indirect force from a varus stress with internal rotation of the tibia stretching of the anterior cruciate ligament and lateral capsule.
Symptoms	Pain on active movement; pain on passive stress; loss of normal knee function; pain on resistive movement; tenderness.
Signs	Point tenderness at the attachment of the anterior cruciate ligament on the tibia; swelling; hemorrhage; possible deformity with third-degree injury; anterolateral instability with second- and third-degree injury; inflammation; ecchymosis; loss of normal knee function.
Special Tests	Assessment of range of motion and ligamentous stability test to include the lateral pivot shift, Slocum test, Hughston test, and flexion–rotation drawer test.
Referral/ Diagnostic Procedure	Refer to an orthopedic surgeon. MRI.
Classification of Injury	First-, second-, and third-degree. See Chapter 1 for classification of sprain injury.

Medical Term	Sprain/Posterolateral instability
Common Term	Same as above
Mechanisms	Indirect force such as hyperextension causing a stretching of the posterior cruciate ligament.
Symptoms	Pain on active movement; pain on passive stress; loss of function; pain on resistive movement; tenderness.
Signs	Swelling; hemorrhage; possible deformity with third degree injury; ecchymosis; instability with second and third degree injury; inflammation; loss of function; posterolateral point tenderness.
Special Tests	Assessment of range of motion and ligamentous stability test including the gravity drawer test, Lachman's test, external rotation–recurvatum test, gravity external rotation test, and posterior drawer test.
Referral/ Diagnostic Procedure	Refer to an orthopedic surgeon.
Classification of Injury	First-, second-, and third-degree. See Chapter 1 for classification of sprain injury.

Medical Term	**Plica irritation**
Common Term	Same as above
Mechanisms	Indirect trauma as with torsion and a foot planted. Overuse such as running.
Symptoms	Painful pseudo–locking after sitting; pain on using stairs or squatting.
Signs	Popping as the knee passes 20° to 30° of flexion while weight bearing; popping is usually over the superior/medial aspect of the patella.
Special Tests	Flex the knee 20° to 30° while weight bearing and palpate for a popping sensation.
Referral/ Diagnostic Procedure	Refer to an orthopedic surgeon.
Classification of Injury	Not applicable

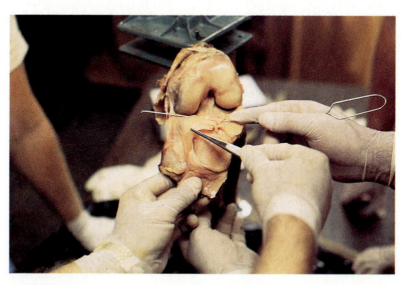

Forceps holding the synovial plica of the knee.

Medical Term	**Knee contusion**
Common Term	Bruised knee
Mechanisms	Direct trauma.
Symptoms	Pain; loss of function; transitory paralysis of knee flexion and extension; tenderness at the site of the trauma.
Signs	Point tenderness; ecchymosis; hematoma formation; inflammation; loss of function.
Special Tests	Not applicable
Referral/ Diagnostic Procedure	Not applicable
Classification of Injury	First-, second-, and third-degree. See Chapter 1 for classification of contusion injury.

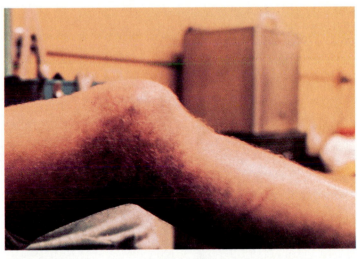

Knee contusion indicated by swelling and ecchymosis.

Medical Term	**Medial meniscal tear**
Common Term	Torn cartilage
Mechanisms	Indirect force applied to the knee, while the foot is planted, causing external rotation of the tibia; hyperflexion; cutting motion; prolonged overuse.
Symptoms	Pain; periodic locking; sensation of the knee "giving way"; possible clicking sensation when going up and down stairs; pain when squatting.
Signs	Medial joint line pain; swelling; possible locking; weakened quadriceps muscle.
Special Tests	McMurry's test; Apley's compression test; modified Apley's compression test; bounce home test. Assessment of range of motion and strength.
Referral/ Diagnostic Procedure	Not applicable
Classification of Injury	Not applicable

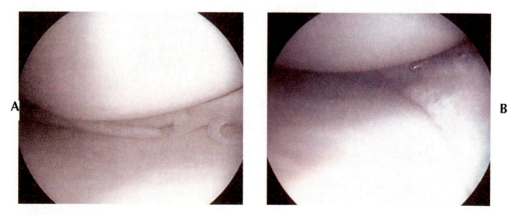

A, Arthroscopic view of torn medial meniscus. **B**, Arthroscopic view of medial meniscus after repair.

Medical Term	**Pes anserine tendinitis**
Common Term	Cyclist's knee
Mechanisms	Overuse as in long-distance running causing repeated microtrauma to the tendon or to the muscle–tendon attachments; degenerative changes in the tendon; weakness of the vastus medialis and excessive genu valgum.
Symptoms	Pain on active knee flexion and extension; pain on passive stretch; reported overuse activity; pain on the medial tibial plateau.
Signs	Swelling over the pes anserine attachment on the tibia; loss of normal knee function; point tenderness at the pes anserine attachment on the tibia; possible crepitus; inflammation.
Special Tests	Assessment of range of motion and strength.
Referral/ Diagnostic Procedure	Refer to an orthopedic surgeon if symptom/signs persist.
Classification of Injury	Not applicable

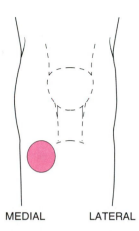

MEDIAL   LATERAL

Area of pain for pes anserine tendinitis.

Medical Term	**Popliteus tendinitis**
Common Term	Same as above
Mechanisms	Overuse, as in long-distance running, causing repeated microtraumas and degenerative changes in the popliteus tendon.
Symptoms	Pain on active movement; loss of normal knee function; reported overuse activity; pain on resistive movement; tenderness; pain on knee flexion; pain in the posterior aspect of the knee.
Signs	Swelling; loss of normal knee function; possible crepitus; inflammation; point tenderness over the posterior aspect of the knee.
Special Tests	Assessment of range of motion and strength.
Referral/ Diagnostic Procedure	Refer to an orthopedic surgeon is symptoms/signs persist.
Classification of Injury	Not applicable

Medical Term	**Patella tendinitis**
Common Term	Jumper's knee
Mechanisms	Overuse, such as in jumping or running, causing repeated microtrauma and degenerative changes in the patella tendon.
Symptoms	Pain on active movement; pain on passive stretch; loss of function; reported overuse activity such as running or jumping; pain on resistive movement; tenderness; pain on knee extension.
Signs	Swelling; loss of function; possible crepitus; possible calcium formation; inflammation; point tenderness over the patella tendon.
Special Tests	Assessment of range of motion and strength.
Referral/ Diagnostic Procedure	Refer to an orthopedic surgeon if symptoms/signs persist.
Classification of Injury	Not applicable

■ SPECIAL TESTS FOR THE KNEE ■

(All tests should be performed bilaterally)

■ TESTS FOR PATELLOFEMORAL CONDITIONS

Q-Angle

The athletic trainer draws a line from the anterior superior iliac spine through the midpoint of the patella. Then the athletic trainer draws a line from the tuberosity of the tibia straight up the middle of the patella, creating an angle. If this angle is greater than 18° to 20°, this can create patellofemoral problems.

Apprehension Test

The athletic trainer places the athlete in a supine position and tells him or her to relax the quadriceps and hamstrings. The athletic trainer then moves the patella laterally, looking for laxity in the joint capsule. This test is used to determine if the patella is subluxing or dislocating laterally. A positive test is indicated by the athlete's apprehension to allow the patella toward the area of the subluxation or dislocation.

Patella Compression Test

The athletic trainer places the athlete in a supine position, places an object under the athlete's knee to put the knee in approximately 20° of flexion, and makes sure the quadriceps and hamstrings are relaxed. The athletic trainer then pushes the patella down into the femoral groove and moves the patella forward and backward, trying to produce a grinding sensation and/or discomfort, which indicates possible pathology on the articular surface of the patella, such as chondromalacia.

Patella Grind Test

The athletic trainer places the athlete in a supine position, places an object under the knee to put the knee in approximately 20° of flexion, and makes sure the quadriceps and hamstrings are relaxed. The athletic trainer then pushes the patella distally and asks the athlete to extend the knee with a contraction of the quadriceps. The athletic trainer should feel for any grinding sensation as the patella moves anteriorly. The movement should be smooth and gliding.

■ TESTS FOR EFFUSION OF THE KNEE

Ballottable Patella Test

The athletic trainer places the athlete in a supine position and asks the athlete to extend the leg as far as possible and relax the quadriceps and hamstrings. The athletic trainer then pushes the patella into the trochlear groove and releases the patella. If the knee has a major effusion, the patella will rebound because the fluid that was forced out from under it on compression moves back under it when it is released. This test is similar to pushing in on a balloon and then releasing the pressure.

Bounce Home Test

This test is used to check for joint swelling, meniscus tears, or loose bodies in the knee. The athletic trainer places the athlete in a supine position, fully flexes the knee, and then passively extends the knee. The knee should move to full extension with a definite end point. If the knee does not move to full extension and has a rubbery–feeling end point, something is restricting its motion. This could be swelling, a torn meniscus, or loose bodies in the knee.

■ TESTS FOR ACTIVE AND RESISTIVE RANGE OF MOTION

Flexion and Extension Test

The athletic trainer places the athlete in a prone or sitting position on a table with the lower leg extended over the end of the table. He or she then instructs the athlete to flex the knee actively through the range of motion (135°) and then extend the leg to full extension (0°). If the athlete can actively flex and extend the knee through the range of motion, the athletic trainer then applies resistance in both flexion and extension. Extension can be tested with the athlete sitting on the end of a table with the knees flexed at 90°, and then move to extension actively and resistively. If the athlete cannot move through the full range of motion actively, then a passive range of motion test should be done.

■ TESTS FOR MENISCUS

McMurry's Test

The athletic trainer places the athlete in a supine position on a table and tells him or her to relax the quadriceps and hamstrings. The athletic trainer grasps the athlete's foot in one hand and places the other hand over the joint line, cupping the joint line, with the index finger over the medial joint line and the thumb over the lateral joint line. The athletic trainer then flexes the knee, and internally and externally rotates the tibia several times to loosen the knee, after which he or she externally rotates the tibia, applies a valgus force at the knee, and slowly extends the knee, feeling for any popping sensation at the joint line (test the medial meniscus). Next, the athletic trainer flexes the knee, internally rotates the tibia, applies a varus force, and slowly extends the knee, feeling for any popping sensation at the joint line (test the lateral meniscus). If positive, this test will produce pain with approximately 20° to 30° of extension as the leg is being extended. This test is not highly accurate.

Apley's Compression Test

The athletic trainer places the athlete in a prone position on a table with the knee flexed at 90° and tells him or her to relax the quadriceps and hamstrings. The athletic trainer applies a downward force while internally and externally rotating the tibia, compressing the proximal end of the tibia against the meniscus and femur. This test is not highly accurate. A positive test produces pain.

Modified Apley's Compression Test

The athletic trainer places the athlete in a supine position on a table and tells him or her to relax the quadriceps and hamstrings. The athletic trainer moves the athlete's knee in flexion and extension while applying a valgus and varus force at the knee joint. This test applies compression to the medial (valgus force) and lateral (varus force) meniscus. This is not a highly accurate test.

■ TESTS FOR LIGAMENT STABILITY (UNIDIRECTIONAL LAXITIES)

Anterior Drawer Test

This test is for straight anterior instability and for testing the anterior cruciate ligament. The athletic trainer places the athlete in a supine position on a table with the knee flexed at 90°. The athletic trainer stabilizes the athlete's foot, places the hand around the proximal end of the tibia, and makes sure the hamstrings are relaxed. He or she then applies an anterior pull on the tibia, looking for a forward shift of the tibia.

Lachman's Test

This test is for straight anterior instability and for testing the anterior cruciate ligament. The athletic trainer places the athlete in a supine position and tells him or her to relax the quadriceps and hamstrings. The athletic trainer grasps the femur with one hand and the proximal tibia with the other hand and flexes the knee to approximately 30°, then stabilizes the femur and applies an anterior pull on the tibia, looking for a forward shift of the tibia and a distinct endpoint.

Posterior Drawer Test

This test is for straight posterior instability and for testing the posterior cruciate ligament. The athlete and athletic trainer are in the same position as for the anterior drawer test, except this time the trainer applies a posterior force against the tibia, looking for a posterior shift of the tibia and a distinct end point.

Gravity Drawer Test

This test is for straight posterior instability and for testing the posterior cruciate ligament. The athletic trainer places the athlete in a supine position, and tells him or her to relax the quadriceps and hamstrings, flexes the hip and knee to 90°, and observes whether there is a posterior subluxation of the tibia on the femur. The heel can be placed in a chair that is placed on the table.

Valgus (Abduction) Stress Test

This test is for straight medial instability and for testing the tibial collateral ligament (medial collateral ligament). The athletic trainer places the athlete in a supine position and tells him or her to relax the quadriceps and hamstrings. The athletic trainer places one hand on the medial side of the distal tibia and the other hand at the lateral joint line. First, with the athlete's knee in full extension, the athletic trainer applies a valgus force to the knee, observing for medial joint laxity, then he or she flexes the knee approximately 30° and repeats the test. Joint line opening in full extension indicates damage to the posterior cruciate ligament. Joint line opening at 30° of flexion indicates damage to the tibial collateral ligament.

Varus (Adduction) Stress Test

This test is for straight lateral instability and for testing the fibular collateral ligament (lateral collateral ligament). The athletic trainer places the athlete in a supine position and tells him or her to relax the quadriceps and hamstrings. The athletic trainer places the athlete in a supine position and tells him or her to relax the quadriceps and hamstrings. The athletic trainer places one hand on the lateral side of the distal fibula and the other hand over the medial joint line. First, with the athlete's knee in full extension, the athletic trainer applies a varus force to the knee, looking for lateral joint laxity. Then he or she flexes the knee approximately 30° and repeats the test. Lateral laxity at 30°

of flexion indicates fibula collateral ligament damage and lateral capsule damage. Joint laxity in full extension indicates fibula collateral ligament damage and posterolateral capsule damage.

■ TESTS FOR LIGAMENT STABILITY (MULTIDIRECTIONAL LAXITIES)

Slocum External Rotation Test

This test is for anteriomedial instability and for testing the anterior cruciate ligament, superficial tibial collateral ligament, and medial and posterior medial capsule. The athletic trainer places the athlete supine on a table, flexes the athlete's knee at 80°, flexes the hip at 45°, sits on the foot for stabilization, and tells the athlete to relax the quadriceps and hamstrings. The athletic trainer places his or her hands behind the proximal tibia and pulls forward on the tibia, noting any rotation of the medial tibial plateau from under the medial femoral condyle, as compared to the other knee. Then an external rotation force is applied to the medial tibial condyle, and the amount of external rotation is noted. After this test has been performed, the athlete's tibia is externally rotated approximately 10°, and the test is repeated. When the middle tibial plateau rotates anteriorly, the test is positive

Valgus (Abduction) Stress Test

This test is performed in the same manner as described for straight medial instabilities with the knee flexed, except that in this test, as the valgus force is applied, the trainer also externally rotates the tibia.

Lateral Pivot Shift

This test is for anterolateral instabilities and for testing the anterior cruciate ligament and lateral structures of the knee. The athletic trainer places the athlete in a supine position on a table and tells him or her to relax the quadriceps and hamstrings. The athletic trainer grasps the heel in one hand and places the other hand over the lateral tibia with the thumb behind the fibular head. The tibia is internally rotated, a valgus force is applied at the knee, and the knee is moved from a full extension to approximately 30° of flexion. At this point, the athletic trainer may feel a subluxation of the lateral aspect of the tibia. There will be a visible, palpable, and audible reduction as the subluxation occurs.

Slocum Test

This test is for anterolateral instability of the knee and for testing the anterior cruciate ligament and lateral structures of the knee. The athletic trainer places the athlete on their side with the uninjured leg flexed at the knee and hip, and permits the hip and knee on the injured leg to fall back. The injured leg is placed in full extension. The athletic trainer grasps the heel of the injured leg in one hand, places the other hand over the lateral femoral condyle and internally rotates the tibia, and applies a valgus force as the knee is flexed to approximately 30°. The athletic trainer should observe the signs as in the lateral pivot shift test.

Hughston Jerk Test

This test is for anterolateral instability of the knee and for testing the anterior cruciate and lateral structures of the knee. The athletic trainer places the athlete in a supine position on a table and tells him or her to relax the quadriceps and hamstrings. The leg is flexed at 90°, the tibia is internally rotated, a valgus force is applied, and the knee is slowly extended. At approximately 30° the athletic trainer should observe the same signs as with the lateral pivot shift test. If the knee is carried to full extension, reduction occurs again.

Flexion–Rotation Drawer Test

This test is for anterolateral instability of the knee and for testing the anterior cruciate and lateral structures of the knee. The athletic trainer places the athlete in a supine position on a table and tells him or her to relax the quadriceps and hamstrings. The leg is held in a neutral position at about 20° of flexion. If the anterior cruciate ligament is torn, the femur will drop posteriorly, due to the weight of the thigh, and externally rotate. This position produces a subluxation position of the lateral tibiofemoral joint. The athletic trainer flexes the knee 10° while applying a downward pressure on the tibia producing a reduction position. The athletic trainer moves the leg back and forth from the starting position to the ending position. This test is a modification of the lateral pivot shift and the Lachman's test.

External Rotation–Recurvatum Test

This test is for posterolateral rotatory instability and for testing the posterolateral ligamentous structures, including the arcuate ligament complex, popliteal tendon, and the fibular collateral ligament. The athletic trainer places the athlete in the supine position on a table and tells him or her to relax the quadriceps and hamstrings. The athletic trainer then picks up the foot of the injured leg and observes the external rotation of the lateral tibia on the femur and any recurvatum associated with this movement.

Gravity External Rotation Test

This test is for posterolateral rotatory instability and for testing the posterolateral ligamentous structures, including the arcuate ligament complex, popliteal tendon, and the fibular collateral ligament. The athletic trainer places the athlete in the supine position on a table, tells him or her to relax the quadriceps and hamstrings, and flexes the athlete's hip and knee to 90°. The athletic trainer then grasps the distal end of the tibia with one hand, places the other hand over the fibula head, externally rotates the tibia, and observes the movement of the fibular head and tuberosity of the tibia from normal.

■ TEST FOR ILIOTIBIAL BAND SYNDROME

Ober's Test

The athlete should lie on the side of their uninvolved leg. Abduct the affected leg as far as possible with the knee flexed at 90° and the hip in a neutral position, then release the leg into adduction. If the iliotibial band is normal, the leg will drop into full adduction. If the iliotibial is tight, the leg will remain in abduction.

Noble Compression Test

The athlete should lie supine on the table with the knee flexed at 90°. The athlete trainer applies pressure with their thumb to the lateral femoral epicondyle and maintain the pressure as the athlete extends their knee. A positive test is pain when the iliotibial band passes over the lateral epicondyle.

■ GENERAL ASSESSMENT TEST FOR JOINT RANGE OF MOTION AND STRENGTH FOR A STRAIN, TENDINITIS, AND TENOSYNO-VITIS

Active Movement

The athlete moves the body part through the range of motion actively, trying to reproduce the pain.

Passive Stretch

The athletic trainer performs a passive stretch of the involved muscle or tendon.

Resistive Movement

The athlete moves the body part through the range of motion while the athletic trainer applies resistance.

■ GENERAL ASSESSMENT TEST FOR RANGE OF MOTION AND LIGAMENTOUS STABILITY FOR A SPRAIN

Active Movement

The athlete moves the joint through the range of motion actively. The athletic trainer should be looking for any limitations in the range of motion.

Passive Movement

If the athlete cannot move the joint through the range of motion actively, then passive range of motion should be done to determine whether the range of motion is blocked due to the athlete's pain, or because some object is blocking the joint.

Resistive Movement

The athlete moves the joint through the range of motion, while the athletic trainer applies resistance.

Passive Stress

The athletic trainer applies stress to the joint to test the integrity of the ligamentous structures of the joint.

LOWER LEG INJURIES AND CONDITIONS

Chapter 16

Acute Anterior Compartment
  Syndrome
Retrocalcaneal Bursitis
Contusion of Lower Leg
Chronic Exercise–Induced
  Compartment Compression
  Syndrome
Fibula Fracture
Fibula Stress Fracture
Tibia Stress Fracture
Tibia Fracture

Tibial Plateau Fracture
Medial Tibial Stress Syndrome
Plantaris Muscle Rupture
General Muscle Spasm
Gastrocnemius Strain
Anterior Talotibial Exostosis
Posterior Talotibial Exostosis
Achilles Tendinitis
Tendo Achilles Rupture
Achilles Tendon Tenosynovitis

Medical Term	Acute anterior compartment syndrome
Common Term	Same as above
Mechanisms	Direct trauma to the anterior compartment of the lower leg, as in being kicked.
Symptoms	Possible loss of ankle dorsiflexors or great toe extension; pain during running; pain on active and resistive dorsiflexion; pain on passive plantar flexion.
Signs	Swelling in the anterior lower leg; tenderness; possible dropped foot; possible loss of sensation in the web of the first and second toe or the dorsum of the foot; pain on passive plantar flexion; pain on active and resistive ankle dorsiflexion and great toe extension; inability to evert the foot; hardness of fascia in the anterior lower leg.
Special Tests	Active and resistive dorsiflexion; passive plantar flexion; check neurologic sensation, check dorsal pedal pulse.
Referral/ Diagnostic Procedure	Refer to an orthopedic surgeon or general surgeon.
Classification of Injury	Not applicable

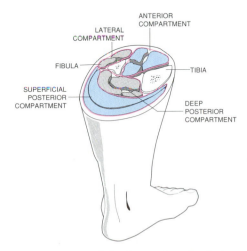

Cross-section of the lower leg depicting the four compartments, including the anterior.

Medical Term	**Retrocalcaneal bursitis**
Common Term	Bursitis
Mechanisms	Overuse as in running; direct trauma as in constant external pressure from footwear.
Symptoms	Pain located near the attachment of the achilles tendon; loss of normal ankle function; tenderness.
Signs	Redness; swelling; loss of normal ankle function; possible calcium formation in chronic cases; inflammation; point tenderness.
Special Tests	Not applicable
Referral/ Diagnostic Procedure	Refer to an orthopedic surgeon if symptoms/signs persist.
Classification of Injury	Not applicable

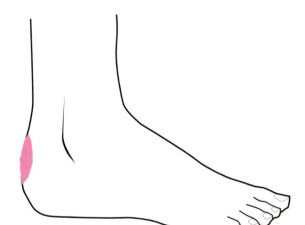

Common tendinitis of the foot and ankle region.

Medical Term	Contusion of lower leg
Common Term	Bruise
Mechanisms	Direct trauma as in being kicked in the leg.
Symptoms	Pain; loss of function; transitory paralysis of the muscles of in the area of the contusion; tenderness in the area of the contusion.
Signs	Point tenderness; ecchymosis; hematoma formation; inflammation; loss of function.
Special Tests	Assessment of range of motion and strength test.
Referral/ Diagnostic Procedure	Refer to a physician if symptoms/signs persist.
Classification of Injury	First-, second-, and third-degree. See Chapter 1 for classification of contusion injury.

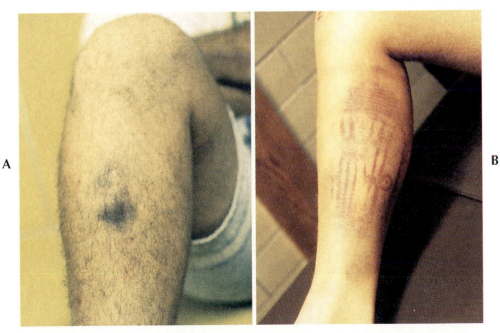

A, Swelling and ecchymosis due to contusion to lower leg. B, Second-degree contusion.

Medical Term	Chronic exercise–induced compartment compression syndrome
Common Term	Same as above
Mechanisms	Extensive running that causes tissue fluid pressure to increase because of the restraints of the fascia and/or bone, adversely compressing muscles, blood vessels, and nerves.
Symptoms	In chronic cases, symptoms include pain and pressure during activity that subsides with rest; possible numbness on the dorsum of the foot; weakness on dorsiflexion and toe extension.
Signs	In acute cases, signs include swelling and loss of ankle function. In chronic cases, signs may include ischemia, loss of function, and swelling.
Special Tests	Check dorsal pedal pulse.
Referral/ Diagnostic Procedure	Refer to an orthopedic surgeon or general surgeon.
Classification of Injury	Not applicable

Medical Term	**Fibula fracture**
Common Term	Broken leg
Mechanisms	Direct trauma as in a blow directly to the fibula; indirect force as in a eversion ankle sprain.
Symptoms	Sudden pain; loss of function; direct and indirect tenderness.
Signs	Loss of function; possible deformity; rapid swelling; direct tenderness; indirect tenderness; possible bony deviation; possible crepitus; possible false motion; delayed ecchymosis; pain on forced eversion; possible inability to bear weight on the leg; pain on compression of upper tibia and fibula.
Special Tests	Forced eversion; compression of the tibia and fibula.
Referral/ Diagnostic Procedure	Refer to an orthopedic surgeon. X–ray.
Classification of Injury	Not applicable

Medical Term	**Fibula stress fracture**
Common Term	Same as above
Mechanisms	Overuse; repeated loading on the bone over a long period of time.
Symptoms	No history of impact or trauma. Increased pain on activity that subsides with rest; possible increase in training reported; tenderness.
Signs	Point tenderness; swelling; loss of function; possible pain on weight bearing; inflammation.
Special Tests	Not applicable
Referral/ Diagnostic Procedure	Refer to an orthopedic surgeon. X–ray, bone scan.
Classification of Injury	Not applicable

Medical Term	Tibia stress fracture
Common Term	Same as above
Mechanisms	Overuse; repeated loading of the bone over a long period of time.
Symptoms	No history of impact or trauma; increased pain upon activity that subsides with rest; possible increase in training reported; tenderness.
Signs	Point tenderness; loss of function; swelling; inflammation; pain on weight bearing.
Special Tests	Not applicable
Referral/ Diagnostic Procedure	Refer to an orthopedic surgeon. X–ray, bone scan.
Classification of Injury	Not applicable

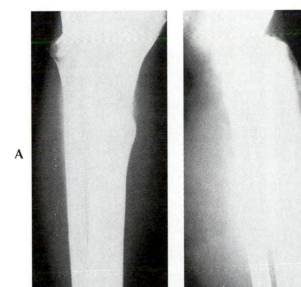

A and **B**, Increase of calcium buildup at area of stress fracture.

Medical Term	Tibia fracture
Common Term	Broken leg
Mechanisms	Direct force applied to the tibia; indirect force as in violent stresses causing forceful adduction or abduction of the knee or torsion as in skiing.
Symptoms	Sudden pain; loss of function; direct and indirect tenderness; inability to bear weight on the leg.
Signs	Loss of function; possible deformity; rapid swelling; direct tenderness; indirect tenderness; possible bony deviation; possible crepitus; possible false motion; delayed ecchymosis; pain on weight bearing.
Special Tests	Not applicable
Referral/ Diagnostic Procedure	Refer to an orthopedic surgeon. X–ray.
Classification of Injury	Not applicable

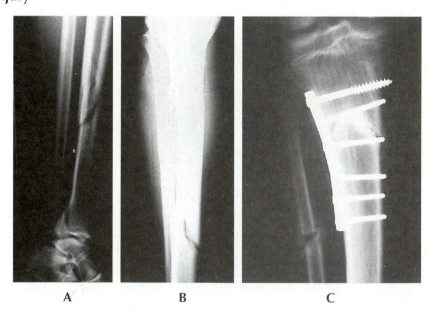

A and B, Fractured tibia. C, Repair of fractured tibia.

Medical Term	**Tibial plateau fracture**
Common Term	Same as above
Mechanisms	Direct force such as axial loading combined with valgus or varus forces; indirect force such as planted foot and rotation of trunk.
Symptoms	Acute pain, unable to move knee joint.
Signs	Swelling; loss of knee function; possible deformity; pain over tibial metaphysis.
Special Tests	Tap test
Referral/ Diagnostic Procedure	Refer to physician for x–ray evaluation; aspiration showing hemarthosis is common.
Classification of Injury	Not applicable

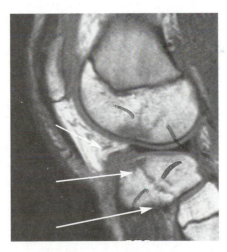

Tibial plateau fracture *(arrows)*.

Medical Term	**Medial tibial stress syndrome**
Common Term	Shin splints
Mechanisms	Predisposing factors such as faulty posture alignment, falling arches, muscle fatigue, overuse, lack of coordination causing injury to the posterior tibialis or toe flexor tendons.
Symptoms	Pain in the anterior leg. *Grade one:* pain after activity; *grade two:* pain before and after activity; *grade three:* pain before, during, and after activity; *grade four:* no participation due to pain; loss of normal ankle function.
Signs	Possible swelling; inflammation; loss of normal ankle function; abnormal gait; pain on active and resistive dorsiflexion; pain on passive stretch of dorsiflexors.
Special Tests	Assessment of range of motion and strength.
Referral/ Diagnostic Procedure	Refer to an orthopedic surgeon if symptoms/signs persist. X–ray, bone scan for stress fracture.
Classification of Injury	First-, second-, or third-degree. See Chapter 1 for classification of strain injury.

Area of pain for medial tibial stress syndrome.

Medical Term	**Plantaris muscle rupture**
Common Term	Tennis leg
Mechanisms	Excessive contraction or stretch of the musculotendinous unit, as in running or jumping; sudden change in direction.
Symptoms	Pain in the lower leg with running or jumping; sudden pain deep in the lower leg; possible pain around the ankle; possible loss of function in severe cases. The athlete describes pain on "push off" that feels like being shot in the back of the leg. Tenderness about 10 inches (25 cm) below the knee laterally or medially.
Signs	Tenderness about 10 inches (25 cm) below the knee laterally or medially; nodule may be palpable in the gastrocnemius area; pain with dorsiflexion of the foot; possible delayed ecchymosis and edema around the ankle; loss of function.
Special Tests	Assessment of range of motion and strength test; Thompson test.
Referral/ Diagnostic Procedure	Refer to an orthopedic surgeon. MRI.
Classification of Injury	Not applicable

Medical Term	**General muscle spasm**
Common Term	Cramp
Mechanisms	Predisposing factors, such as lack of electrolytes, fluid loss, muscle fatigue or reflex to direct trauma as in a contusion.
Symptoms	Pain; loss of normal muscle function; tenderness.
Signs	Involuntary muscle contraction; loss of normal muscle function; direct tenderness over the area of the spasm.
Special Tests	Not applicable
Referral/ Diagnostic Procedure	Refer to a physician if symptoms/signs persist.
Classification of Injury	Not applicable

Medical Term	Gastrocnemius strain
Common Term	Same as above
Mechanisms	Overuse as in running; indirect trauma to the musculo-tendinous unit due to excessive contraction or stretching; predisposing muscle fatigue.
Symptoms	Pain increased with active and resistive ankle plantar flexion; pain on passive stretch; loss of ankle plantar flexion; possible snapping sound heard when the injury occurs; muscle fatigue before injury; tenderness; muscle tightness before injury. The athlete reports a pain that feels like being shot in the leg.
Signs	Muscle spasm; swelling; ecchymosis; point tenderness; loss of strength; loss of ankle plantar flexion; hematoma formation and defect in the musculotendinous unit with third-degree injury; inflammation.
Special Tests	Assessment of range of motion and strength test.
Referral/ Diagnostic Procedure	Active and resistive plantar flexion; passive dorsiflexion.
Classification of Injury	First-, second-, and third-degree. See Chapter 1 for classification of strain injury.

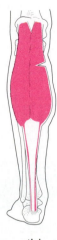

Location of possible tear in gas-trocnemius muscle due to strain.

Medical Term	Anterior talotibial exostosis
Common Term	Same as above
Mechanisms	Repetitive extreme dorsiflexion causing contact between the talus and the tibia; the repetition causes inflammation and irritation, which eventually leads to bone formation.
Symptoms	Pain across the ankle joint; pain in the ankle during "push off" phase of running or the "drive phase" of blocking in football; pain on forceful manual dorsiflexion; tenderness over the dorsum of the ankle at the joint of the talus and tibia. The athlete states that he or she cannot run full speed.
Signs	Point tenderness at the dome of the talus; mild loss of function of the ankle joint; inability to "drive off" a planted foot; spurs that are visible on x–ray.
Special Tests	Forced dorsiflexion of the ankle.
Referral/ Diagnostic Procedure	Refer to an orthopedic surgeon. X–ray.
Classification of Injury	Not applicable

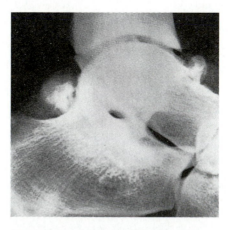

Impingement caused by exostosis
on the anterior area of the talus as
indicated by bony fragments.

Medical Term	**Posterior talotibial exostosis**
Common Term	Bony spur
Mechanisms	Repetitive extreme plantar flexion that causes traction on the attachment of the joint capsule, resulting in microscopic bleeding and eventually spur formation.
Symptoms	Pain in the posterior aspect of the ankle; pain on forced plantar flexion; loss of normal ankle function; tenderness. The athlete states that he or she cannot run full speed.
Signs	Tenderness in the posterior aspect of the ankle; pain on forced plantar flexion; loss of normal ankle function; spurs that show on x–ray.
Special Tests	Forced plantar flexion.
Referral/ Diagnostic Procedure	Refer to an orthopedic surgeon. X–ray.
Classification of Injury	Not applicable

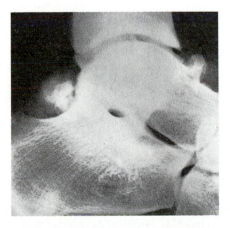

Impingement caused by exostosis on the posterior area of the talus and calcaneus as indicated by bony fragments.

Medical Term	Achilles tendinitis
Common Term	Same as above
Mechanisms	Overuse; repeated microtrauma to the achilles tendon or to the muscle–tendon attachments; degenerative changes in the tendon.
Symptoms	Pain on active and resistive movements; pain on passive stretch; loss of normal ankle function; overuse activity; tenderness.
Signs	Swelling; loss of normal ankle function; possible crepitus; inflammation; point tenderness.
Special Tests	Assessment of range of motion and strength.
Referral/ Diagnostic Procedure	Refer to an orthopedic surgeon if symptoms/signs persist.
Classification of Injury	Not applicable

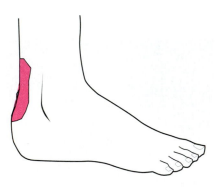

Area of pain for achilles tendinitis.

Medical Term	**Tendo achilles rupture**
Common Term	Same as above
Mechanisms	Strenuous games requiring rising on the toes. Indirect trauma occurring during push–off phase when the knee is extended; following abrupt dorsiflexion of the foot, or occurring when jumping from a height.
Symptoms	Sudden severe pain in the posterior lower leg; possible snapping sound heard when the injury occurs; loss of function.
Signs	Swelling; ecchymosis; defect in the achilles tendon; loss of ankle plantar flexion; inability to rise on the toes.
Special Tests	Thompson test.
Referral/ Diagnostic Procedure	Refer to an orthopedic surgeon.
Classification of Injury	Not applicable

Medical Term	**Achilles tendon tenosynovitis**
Common Term	Same as above
Mechanisms	Indirect trauma causing repeated microtrauma as in long-distance running; degenerative changes; inflammation of sheath covering a tendon.
Symptoms	Pain on active and resistive movements; pain on passive stretch; loss of normal ankle function.
Signs	Swelling; thickening of tendon in chronic cases; snowball crepitus; inflammation.
Special Tests	Assessment of range of motion and strength test.
Referral/ Diagnostic Procedure	Refer to an orthopedic surgeon. MRI.
Classification of Injury	Not applicable

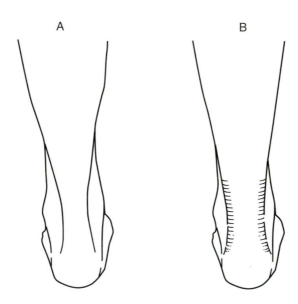

A, Normal achilles tendon. **B,** Noted thickening of the achilles tendon affected by tenosynovitis.

■ TESTS FOR EVALUATION OF INJURIES TO THE ■ LOWER LEG AREA

(All tests should be performed bilaterally)

■ GENERAL ASSESSMENT FOR RANGE OF MOTION AND STRENGTH FOR STRAIN, TENDINITIS, AND TENOSYNOVITIS

Active Movement

The athlete moves the body part through the range of motion actively, trying to reproduce the pain.

Passive Stretch

The athletic trainer performs a passive stretch of the involved muscle or tendon.

Resistive Movement

The athlete moves the body part through the range of motion while the athletic trainer applies resistance.

■ GENERAL ASSESSMENT TEST FOR RANGE OF MOTION AND LIGAMENTOUS STABILITY FOR A SPRAIN

Active Movement

The athlete moves the joint through the range of motion actively. The athletic trainer should be looking for any limitations in the range of motion.

Passive Movement

If the athlete cannot move the joint through the range of motion actively, then passive range of motion should be done to determine whether the range of motion is blocked due to the athlete's pain, or because some object is blocking the joint.

Resistive Movement

The athlete moves the joint through the range of motion, while the athletic trainer applies resistance.

Passive Stress

The athletic trainer applies stress to the joint to test the integrity of the ligamentous structures of the joint.

ANKLE INJURIES AND CONDITIONS

Chapter 17

Medical Term	Tibia chondral/osteochondral fracture
Common Term	Same as above
Mechanisms	Excessive forcible inversion and plantar flexion or eversion and dorsiflexion.
Symptoms	Sudden pain; loss of normal ankle function; direct and indirect tenderness; pain on weight bearing.
Signs	Loss of normal ankle function; possible deformity; rapid swelling; direct tenderness; indirect tenderness; possible bony deviations; possible crepitus; delayed ecchymosis; tenderness over anterolateral confluence of the tibia, fibula, and talus (superolateral); tenderness over the superomedial side of the foot; pain on weight bearing.
Special Tests	Not applicable
Referral/ Diagnostic Procedure	Refer to an orthopedic surgeon. MRI, x–ray.
Classification of Injury	Not applicable

Medical Term   Epiphyseal plate fracture of the distal tibia

Common Term   Not applicable

Mechanisms   Direct trauma to the tibia; indirect trauma as in an excessive compression force or severe torsion in the area of an epiphyseal plate, usually in individuals 10 to 16 years of age.

Symptoms   Sudden pain; loss of normal ankle function; direct and indirect tenderness.

Signs   Loss of normal ankle function; possible deformity; rapid swelling; direct tenderness; indirect tenderness; possible bony deviation; possible crepitus; possible false joint motion; delayed ecchymosis.

Special Tests   Not applicable

Referral/ Diagnostic Procedure   Refer to an orthopedic surgeon. X–ray.

Classification of Injury   See Chapter 1 for classification of epiphyseal plate injury.

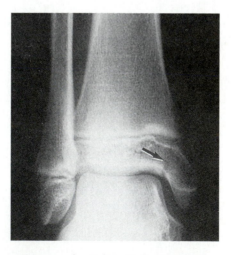

AP view of a Salter III fracture of the distal tibia. Fracture line extends into the articular surface of the tibia *(arrow)*.

Medical Term	**Anterior ankle luxation**
Common Term	Dislocated ankle
Mechanisms	Indirect trauma causing forced dorsiflexion of the foot or a fall upon the heel with the foot in dorsiflexion.
Symptoms	Sudden pain; loss of normal ankle function.
Signs	Marked deformity; loss of normal ankle function; swelling; point tenderness; shortened heel; forefoot lengthened; foot is fixed in dorsiflexion; prominent tibia and fibula.
Special Tests	Check posterior tibial artery and dorsal pedal artery for pulse.
Referral/ Diagnostic Procedure	Refer to an orthopedic surgeon. X– ray.
Classification of Injury	Not applicable

Medical Term	**Posterior ankle luxation**
Common Term	Dislocated ankle
Mechanisms	Indirect force applied to the posterior aspect of the lower leg when the foot is in a plantar flexed position.
Symptoms	Sudden pain; loss of normal ankle function.
Signs	Marked deformity; loss of normal ankle function; swelling; point tenderness; lack of dorsiflexion; lengthened heel; shortened forefoot. The distal end of the tibia and fibula can be palpated in the front of the ankle.
Special Tests	Check the posterior tibial artery and the dorsal pedal artery for pulse.
Referral/ Diagnostic Procedure	Refer to an orthopedic surgeon. X–ray.
Classification of Injury	Not applicable

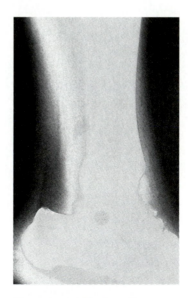

Posterior ankle luxation.

Medical Term	Superior ankle luxation
Common Term	Dislocated ankle
Mechanisms	Indirect trauma forcing the calcaneus and talus upward, as in landing on the foot from a fall.
Symptoms	Sudden pain; loss of normal ankle function.
Signs	Marked deformity; loss of normal ankle function; swelling; point tenderness; spreading of the tibia and fibula malleoli; heel near one or both malleoli.
Special Tests	Check posterior tibial artery and dorsal pedal artery for pulse.
Referral/ Diagnostic Procedure	Refer to an orthopedic surgeon. X–ray.
Classification of Injury	Not applicable

Medical Term	**Peroneal tendon luxation**
Common Term	Same as above
Mechanisms	Direct trauma to the back of the lateral malleolus while the peroneal tendon is taut in dorsiflexion and eversion; predisposing shallow peroneal groove.
Symptoms	Pain; snapping sensation behind the lateral malleolus; ankle weakness; tenderness.
Signs	Luxation of the tendon on resistive dorsiflexion and eversion.
Special Tests	Active, passive, resistive dorsiflexion and eversion.
Referral/ Diagnostic Procedure	Refer to an orthopedic surgeon if symptoms/signs persist.
Classification of Injury	Not applicable

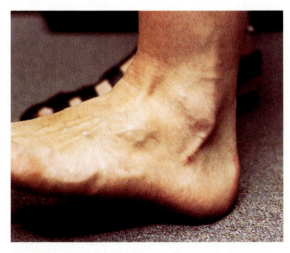

Luxation of the peroneal tendon over the lateral malleolus.

Medical Term	**Eversion ankle sprain**
Common Term	Sprained ankle
Mechanisms	Indirect trauma forcing the ankle into eversion stretching of the medial ligamentous structure of the ankle.
Symptoms	Pain on active and resistive movement; pain on passive stress test; loss of normal ankle function; tenderness over the medial aspect of the ankle.
Signs	Point tenderness over the medial ligamentous structure of the ankle; swelling; hemorrhage; possible deformity with third-degree injury; ecchymosis; possible instability with second- and third-degree injury; inflammation.
Special Tests	Palpate the fibula for a fracture; assessment of range of motion and ligamentous stability; perform an eversion stress test; anterior/posterior drawer test.
Referral/ Diagnostic Procedure	Refer to an orthopedic surgeon. X–ray.
Classification of Injury	First-, second-, and third-degree. See Chapter 1 for classification of sprain injury.

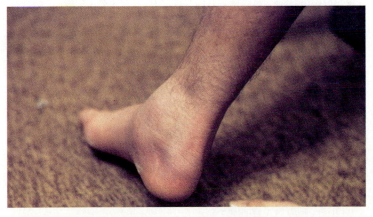

Eversion sprain of the ankle.

Medical Term	**Inversion ankle sprain**
Common Term	Sprained ankle
Mechanisms	Indirect trauma forcing the ankle into inversion stretching of the lateral ligamentous structure of the ankle.
Symptoms	Pain on active and resistive movement; pain on passive stress; loss of normal ankle function; tenderness.
Signs	Point tenderness over the lateral ligamentous structures involved; swelling; hemorrhage; possible deformity with third-degree injury; ecchymosis; instability with second- and third-degree injury; inflammation.
Special Tests	Assessment of range of motion and ligamentous stability; inversion stress test; anterior/posterior drawer test; palpate for fracture of the fibula.
Referral/ Diagnostic Procedure	Refer to an orthopedic surgeon. X–ray.
Classification of Injury	First-, second-, and third-degree. See Chapter 1 for classification of sprain injury.

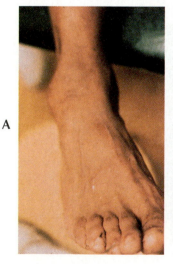 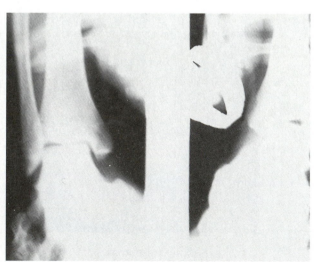

A, First-degree inversion ankle sprain. B, Stress x-ray of inversion ankle sprain.

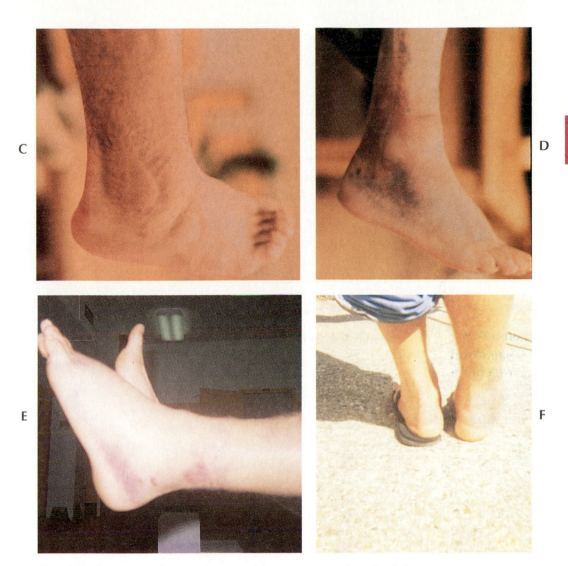

C and **D**, Second-degree inversion ankle sprain. **E** and **F**, Third-degree inversion ankle sprain.

Medical Term	Peroneal tendon tendinitis
Common Term	Same as above
Mechanisms	Indirect trauma as in long-distance running causing repeated microtrauma to the tendon itself or to the musculotendon attachments.
Symptoms	Pain on active and resistive eversion and plantar flexion movements; pain on passive stretch; loss of normal ankle function; overuse activity; tenderness.
Signs	Swelling; loss of normal ankle function on eversion and plantar flexion movements; possible crepitus; possible calcium formation; inflammation; point tenderness over the peroneal tendon.
Special Tests	Assessment of range of motion and strength test.
Referral/ Diagnostic Procedure	Refer to an orthopedic surgeon if symptoms/signs persist.
Classification of Injury	Not applicable

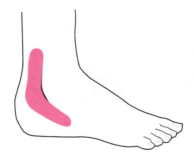

Area of pain for peroneal tendinitis.

TESTS FOR EVALUATION OF INJURIES TO THE ANKLE AREA

(All tests should be performed bilaterally)

GENERAL ASSESSMENT FOR RANGE OF MOTION AND STRENGTH FOR STRAIN, TENDINITIS, AND TENOSYNOVITIS

Active Movement

The athlete moves the body part through the range of motion actively, trying to reproduce the pain.

Passive Stretch

The athletic trainer performs a passive stretch of the involved muscle or tendon.

Resistive Movement

The athlete moves the body part through the range of motion while the athletic trainer applies resistance.

GENERAL ASSESSMENT TEST FOR RANGE OF MOTION AND LIGAMENTOUS STABILITY FOR A SPRAIN

Active Movement

The athlete moves the joint through the range of motion actively. The athletic trainer should be looking for any limitations in the range of motion.

Passive Movement

If the athlete cannot move the joint through the range of motion actively, then passive range of motion should be done to determine whether the range of motion is blocked due to the athlete's pain, or because some object is blocking the joint.

Resistive Movement

The athlete moves the joint through the range of motion, while the athletic trainer applies resistance.

Passive Stress

The athletic trainer applies stress to the joint to test the integrity of the ligamentous structures of the joint.

■ SPECIAL TESTS FOR THE ANKLE

Anterior Drawer Test

The athletic trainer grasps the athlete's heel with one hand and places the other hand in the front of the lower leg at the distal aspect of the tibia and fibula. Then the athletic trainer pulls forward on the heel. If the foot slips forward, there may be ligamentous instability to the ankle. Perform this test bilaterally. Check for distinct end point.

Posterior Drawer Test

The athletic trainer grasps the athlete's lower leg with one hand and the athlete's heel with the other hand. The athletic trainer then pushes the foot in a posterior movement. If the foot moves posteriorly, there may be instability to the ligamentous structure of the ankle. Perform this test bilaterally. Check for distinct end point.

Inversion Stress Test (Talar Tilt Test)

The athletic trainer grasps the athlete's heel in one hand while stabilizing the lower leg with the other hand and moves the athlete's foot into inversion. Abnormal inversion indicates possible ligamentous instability to the lateral ligaments of the ankle. Perform this test bilaterally. Check for distinct end point.

Eversion Stress Test (Talar Tilt Test)

The athletic trainer grasps the athlete's heel in one hand while stabilizing the lower leg with the other hand and moves the foot into eversion. Abnormal eversion indicates possible ligamentous instability to the lateral ligaments of the ankle. Perform this test bilaterally. Check for distinct end point.

FOOT INJURIES AND CONDITIONS

Chapter 18

Sever's Disease

Bulla

Callus

Callus Durum

Callus Molle

Foot Contusion

Heel Contusion

Calcaneus Exostoses

Jones' Fracture

Metatarsal Fracture

Os Callis Fracture

Phalangeal Fracture

Metatarsal Stress Fracture

Tarsal Fracture

Hallicus Ridigus

Hallus Valgus

Hammer Toe

Heel Spur

Subungual Hematoma

Phalangeal Luxation

Metatarsalgia

Morton's Syndrome

Pes Cavus Foot

Pes Planus Foot

Plantar Fascitis

Plantar Neuroma/Interdigital
  Neuroma

Sesamoiditis

Anterior Metatarsal Arch Sprain

Static Arch Sprain

Traumatic Arch Sprain

Great Toe Sprain

Tarsal Tunnel Syndrome

Unguis Incarnates

Verruca Plantaris

Medical Term	Sever's disease
Common Term	Heel pain (apophysitis)
Mechanisms	Caused by stress of the achilles tendon on the apophysis of the calcaneus; common in individuals 10 to 16 years of age.
Symptoms	Pain at the back of the heel; point tenderness; pain of walking and running.
Signs	Occasional swelling at the back of the heel; tightness in the achilles tendon; pain on weight bearing; tenderness; loss of function.
Special Tests	Check for tightness of the achilles tendon.
Referral/ Diagnostic Procedure	Refer to an orthopedic surgeon.
Classification of Injury	Not applicable

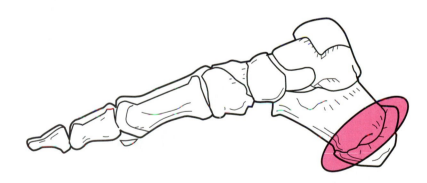

Area of inflammation of the apophyseal plate.

Medical Term	**Bulla**
Common Term	Blister
Mechanisms	Friction caused by improper fitting shoes or excessive training. Usually occurs on the ball of the foot, the great toe, or the heel.
Symptoms	Pain; burning sensation.
Signs	Inflammation; fluid accumulation in intraepidermal slits (fluid may be clear or bloody). Infection can result if the condition is not properly treated.
Special Tests	Not applicable
Referral/ Diagnostic Procedure	Refer to a physician if infected.
Classification of Injury	Not applicable

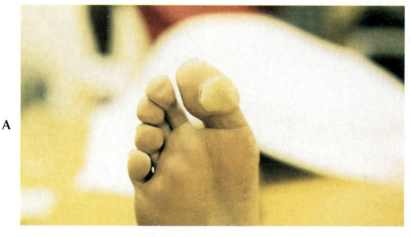

A

A, Open bulla on the great toe.

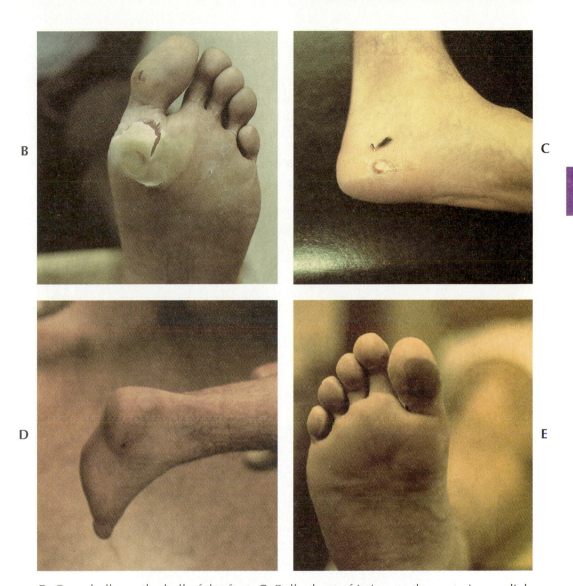

B, Open bulla on the ball of the foot. **C**, Bulla due to friction on the posterior medial heel. **D**, Closed bulla on the posterior aspect of the heel. **E**, Closed bulla on the great toe containing blood.

Medical Term	Callus
Common Term	Same as above
Mechanisms	Friction caused increased activity, such as changing directions when running in basketball, or wearing shoes that are too short or too tight.
Symptoms	Pain due to the loss of elasticity and of the cushioning effect of the fatty layer.
Signs	Thickness of the epidermal skin layer; possible appearance of cracks; possible blister formation under the callus.
Special Tests	Not applicable
Referral/ Diagnostic Procedure	Not applicable
Classification of Injury	Not applicable

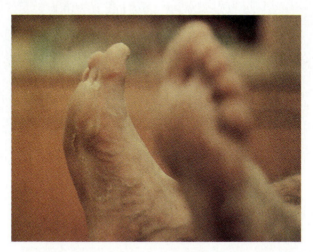

Excessive skin buildup on the ball of the foot and great toe due to friction.

Medical Term	Callus durum
Common Term	Hard corn
Mechanisms	Friction; improperly fitting shoes.
Symptoms	Pain; inability to function in activity due to pain in the area of the corn; tenderness over the area of the corn.
Signs	Inflammation; thickening of soft tissue on the dorsum of the toe; point tenderness; redness.
Special Tests	Not applicable
Referral/ Diagnostic Procedure	Not applicable
Classification of Injury	Not applicable

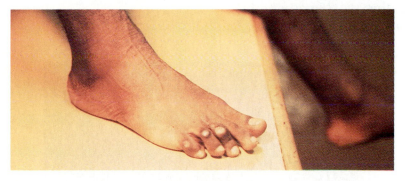

Hard corn on the fifth toe (third and fourth toes have calluses).

Medical Term	Callus molle
Common Term	Soft corn
Mechanisms	Wearing narrow shoes that cause excessive pressure; excessive foot perspiration.
Symptoms	Pain between the toes, usually fourth and fifth; loss of function in severe cases; tenderness.
Signs	Inflammation; circular area of thickened, white, macerated skin, usually between fourth and fifth toes; loss of the ability to run in severe cases; point tenderness at the site of the corn.
Special Tests	Not applicable
Referral/ Diagnostic Procedure	Not applicable
Classification of Injury	Not applicable

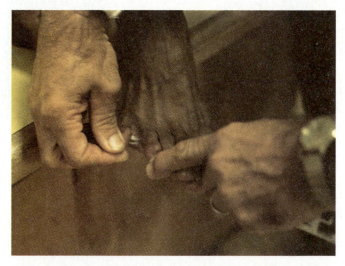

White area on medial side of the fifth toe is a soft corn.

Medical Term	Foot contusion
Common Term	Bruised foot
Mechanisms	Direct trauma.
Symptoms	Pain; loss of locomotion; tenderness.
Signs	Point tenderness; ecchymosis; edema; inflammation; loss of locomotion.
Special Tests	Not applicable
Referral/ Diagnostic Procedure	Not applicable
Classification of Injury	First-, second-, and third-degree. See Chapter 1 for classification of contusion injury.

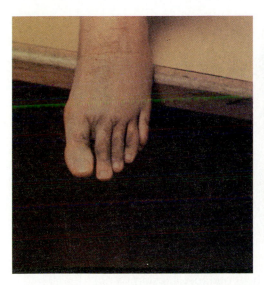 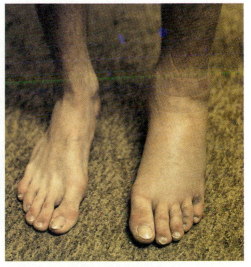

A and **B**, Swelling and ecchymosis of the foot due to contusion.

Medical Term	**Heel contusion**
Common Term	Stone bruise
Mechanisms	Direct trauma, as in a fall from a height or jumping.
Symptoms	Limited ability to function; tenderness on the plantar surface of the foot under the calcaneus.
Signs	Point tenderness on the plantar surface of the foot under the calcaneus; possible ecchymosis; hematoma formation; inflammation; inability to bear weight.
Special Tests	Not applicable
Referral/ Diagnostic Procedure	Not applicable
Classification of Injury	First-, second-, and third-degree. See Chapter 1 for classification of contusion injury.

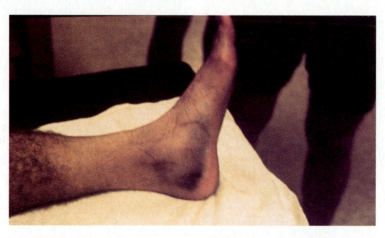

Swelling and ecchymosis of the heel due to contusion.

Medical Term	**Calcaneus exostoses**
Common Term	Spurs
Mechanisms	Repetition of direct trauma to the plantar surface of the calcaneus; indirect causes are heredity, obesity, joint impingement, poor mechanics of walking or running, poorly fitted shoes.
Symptoms	Pain and tenderness on the plantar surface of the calcaneus; loss of the ability to weight bear, as in running and jumping, in severe cases.
Signs	Bony overgrowth at the site of irritation, seen on x–ray; loss of function in severe cases; point tenderness.
Special Tests	Not applicable
Referral/ Diagnostic Procedure	Refer to an orthopedic surgeon. X–ray.
Classification of Injury	Not applicable

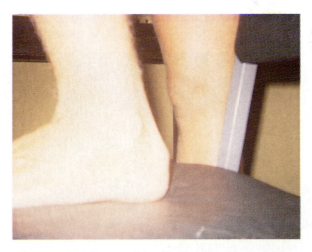

Abnormal contour of the heel at the area of the achilles tendon attachment, indicating exostoses of the calcaneus.

Medical Term	Jones' fracture
Common Term	Fifth metatarsal fracture
Mechanisms	Indirect forces from inversion and plantar flexion of the foot.
Symptoms	Sudden pain at the base of the fifth metatarsal; loss of normal ankle motion; direct and indirect tenderness at the site of the fracture; inability to bear weight on the foot.
Signs	Loss of function; possible deformity; rapid swelling; direct tenderness over the base of the fifth metatarsal; indirect tenderness; possible bony deviation; possible crepitus; possible false joint motion; delayed ecchymosis; inability to bear weight on the foot.
Special Tests	Not applicable
Referral/ Diagnostic Procedure	Refer to an orthopedic surgeon. X–ray.
Classification of Injury	Not applicable

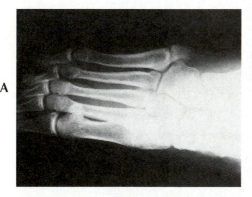 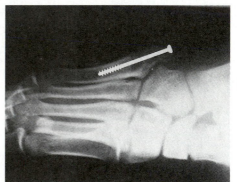

A, Fracture at the base of the fifth metatarsal. **B**, Repair of fracture.

Medical Term	Metatarsal fracture
Common Term	Same as above
Mechanisms	Direct trauma, as being stepped on by another player.
Symptoms	Sudden pain at the site of the fracture, loss of function; direct and indirect tenderness; inability to bear weight on the foot.
Signs	Possible deformity; rapid swelling; direct tenderness at the site of the fracture; indirect tenderness; possible bony deviation; possible crepitus; possible false joint motion; delayed ecchymosis; inability to bear weight on the foot.
Special Tests	Not applicable
Referral/ Diagnostic Procedure	Refer to an orthopedic surgeon. X–ray.
Classification of Injury	Not applicable

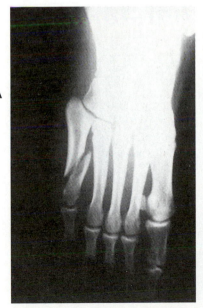 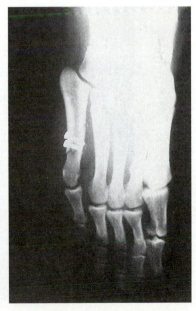

A, Fracture of the shaft of the fifth metatarsal. **B**, Repair of fracture.

Medical Term	Os calis fracture
Common Term	Broken heel bone
Mechanisms	Direct trauma as in a fall or jump from a height.
Symptoms	Sudden pain; loss of function; direct and indirect tenderness; inability to bear weight on the foot.
Signs	Loss of function; possible deformity; rapid swelling; direct tenderness at the site of the fracture; indirect tenderness; possible bony deviation, such as a flattened or widened heel; possible false joint motion; delayed ecchymosis; inability to bear weight on the foot.
Special Tests	Not applicable
Referral/ Diagnostic Procedure	Refer to an orthopedic surgeon. X–ray.
Classification of Injury	Not applicable

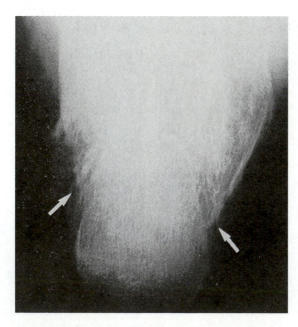

Fracture of calcaneal body *(arrows)*, axial view.

Medical Term	**Phalangeal fracture**
Common Term	Broken toe
Mechanisms	Direct trauma as in kicking an object or stubbing toe.
Symptoms	Sudden pain; loss of foot function; direct and indirect tenderness; abnormal gait.
Signs	Loss of foot function; possible deformity; rapid swelling; direct tenderness; indirect tenderness; possible bony deviation; possible crepitus; possible false joint motion; delayed ecchymosis; abnormal gait.
Special Tests	Not applicable
Referral/ Diagnostic Procedure	Refer to an orthopedic surgeon. X–ray.
Classification of Injury	Not applicable

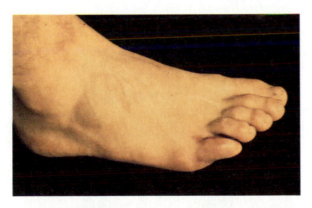

Swelling of the fifth phalange indicating fracture.

Medical Term	**Metatarsal stress fracture**
Common Term	March fracture
Mechanisms	Indirect trauma from overuse as in repeated loading of the bone over a long period of time.
Symptoms	Pain over the affected bone during activity; pain on movement of the metatarsal; reported increase in the athlete's training routine; pain subsides with rest; loss of function; abnormal weight bearing or gait.
Signs	Direct and indirect tenderness at the fracture site; swelling; redness on dorsal aspect over the metatarsal; abnormal weight bearing or gait.
Special Tests	Not applicable
Referral/ Diagnostic Procedure	Refer to an orthopedic surgeon. X–ray; bone scan.
Classification of Injury	Not applicable

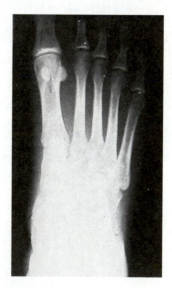

X-ray stress fracture of the
fourth metatarsal.

Medical Term	Tarsal fracture
Common Term	Broken foot
Mechanisms	Direct trauma as in a blow to the foot by another player; indirect trauma from forced dorsiflexion of the foot, transmitting the force upward from the forefoot.
Symptoms	Sudden pain; loss of normal foot function; direct and indirect tenderness; inability to bear weight on the foot.
Signs	Loss of normal foot function; possible deformity; rapid swelling; direct tenderness; indirect tenderness; possible bony deviation; possible crepitus; possible false joint motion; delayed ecchymosis; inability to bear weight on the foot.
Special Tests	Not applicable
Referral/ Diagnostic Procedure	Refer to an orthopedic surgeon. X–ray.
Classification of Injury	Not applicable

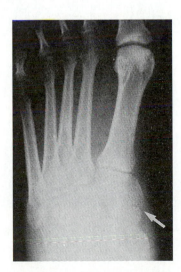

The first cuneiform fracture can be easily seen *(arrow)*, but the metatarsal bases are overlapped in this view.

Medical Term   Hallicus rigidus

Common Term   Same as above

Mechanisms   Fusion or partial fusion of the first metatarsophalangeal joint due to arthritic changes.

Symptoms   Pain; loss of the ability to push off; tenderness of the first metatarsophalangeal joint.

Signs   Loss of ability to push off; direct tenderness of the first metatarsophalangeal joint; inability to extend the great toe; abnormal gait.

Special Tests   Not applicable

Referral/ Diagnostic Procedure   Not applicable

Classification of Injury   Not applicable

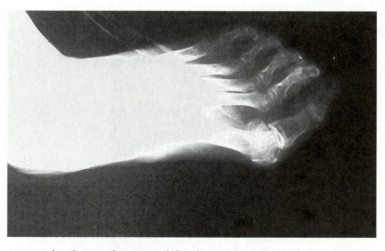

X-ray of arthritic changes of the first metatarsophalangeal joint causing fusion or partial fusion.

Medical Term	Hallus valgus
Common Term	Bunion
Mechanisms	Congenital; indirect causes of wearing shoes too short and too narrow over a long period of time.
Symptoms	Pain over the first metatarsophalangeal joint; difficulty in wearing new footwear; loss of function in severe cases; tenderness; abnormal gait.
Signs	Point tenderness at the first metatarsophalangeal joint; loss of function in severe cases; abnormal gait; angular deformity at the first metatarsophalangeal joint; thick walled bursa over medial prominence of the first metatarsophalangeal joint; swelling; inflammation.
Special Tests	Not applicable
Referral/ Diagnostic Procedure	Not applicable
Classification of Injury	Not applicable

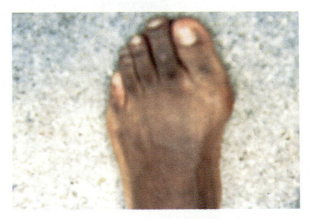

Angular deformity (valgus) at the first metatarsophalangeal joint indicating a bunion.

Medical Term	**Hammer toe**
Common Term	Same as above
Mechanisms	Congenital; wearing shoes too short over a long period of time; intrinsic and extrinsic muscle contracture.
Symptoms	Pain from callus or corns that have formed on the top of the toes because of friction.
Signs	Obvious "hump" or "head of hammer" appearance on the toes; flexion of the distal interphalangeal joint; callus on the top of the toes; possible corns on the tops of the toes.
Special Tests	Not applicable
Referral/ Diagnostic Procedure	Not applicable
Classification of Injury	Not applicable

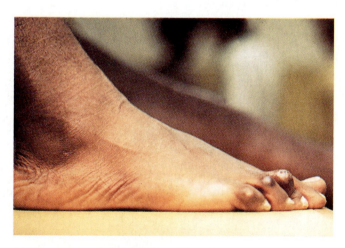

Hammer toe of the third and fourth toes.

Medical Term	**Heel spur**
Common Term	Same as above
Mechanisms	Unknown; may be traumatic or postural as in arch sprain; or spurs may result from repeated trauma to the heel. They are associated with plantar fasciitis.
Symptoms	Pain on the anteromedial aspect of the calcaneum when standing, walking, or running; loss of function; tenderness. The athlete complains of "sticking pain" on the bottom of the foot that causes an abnormal gait.
Signs	Point tenderness over the attachment of the plantar fascia at the calcaneus; loss of function; abnormal gait.
Special Tests	Not applicable
Referral/ Diagnostic Procedure	Refer to an orthopedic surgeon. X–ray to observe calcification at the plantar fascia insertion on the calcaneus.
Classification of Injury	Not applicable

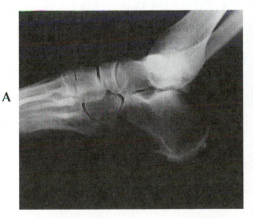
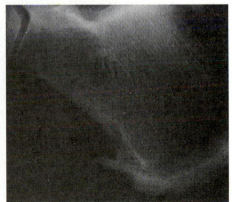

A and B, X-ray of heel spur on the calcaneus.

Medical Term	**Subungual hematoma**
Common Term	Black nail
Mechanisms	Direct trauma to the toenail; wearing shoes too narrow; leaving nails too long; pressing of the nails against the front of the shoe repetitively.
Symptoms	Throbbing pain; tenderness; possible loss of function; possible abnormal gait.
Signs	Point tenderness; possible loss of function of the great toe; possible abnormal gait; blood under the nail.
Special Tests	Not applicable
Referral/ Diagnostic Procedure	Drill the nail to relieve pressure.
Classification of Injury	Not applicable

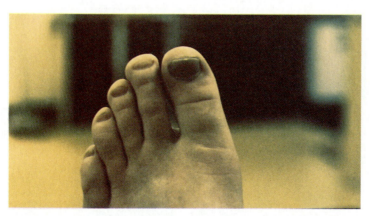

Blood under the nail of the great toe due to direct trauma.

Medical Term	**Phalangeal luxation**
Common Term	Dislocated toe
Mechanisms	Indirect trauma, as in kicking an object or stubbing the toe.
Symptoms	Pain; inability to bear weight on the foot.
Signs	Marked deformity; loss of toe flexion or extension; swelling; point tenderness; ecchymosis; inability to bear weight on the foot.
Special Tests	Not applicable
Referral/ Diagnostic Procedure	Refer to an orthopedic surgeon. X–ray.
Classification of Injury	Not applicable

Medical Term	Metatarsalgia
Common Term	Same as above
Mechanisms	Fallen metatarsal arch.
Symptoms	Pain in the metatarsal, usually beneath the middle metatarsal heads due to depression of the metatarsal arch.
Signs	Callus formation over the area of pain; possible abnormal gait; point tenderness.
Special Tests	Not applicable
Referral/ Diagnostic Procedure	Not applicable
Classification of Injury	Not applicable

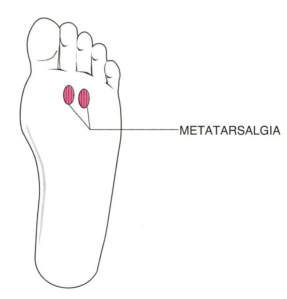

Areas of pain for metatarsalgia.

Medical Term	**Morton's syndrome**
Common Term	Morton's foot
Mechanisms	Short first metatarsal causing more weight bearing through the second toe; hypermobility between the first and second proximal metatarsal joints.
Symptoms	Swelling, pain.
Signs	Overpronation of the forefoot; callus formation in the area of pain; point tenderness; possible abnormal gait.
Special Tests	Not applicable
Referral/ Diagnostic Procedure	Refer to an orthopedic surgeon. Orthosis in the shoes may help the pain.
Classification of Injury	Not applicable

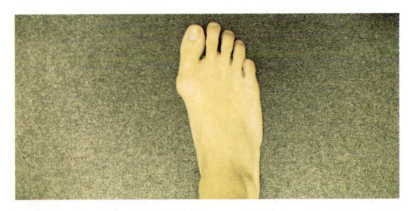

Morton's syndrome indicated by short first metatarsal (second toe longer than first). Also notice bunion on medial side of foot.

Medical Term	**Pes cavus foot**
Common Term	High arch foot
Mechanisms	Congenital, idiopathic, or due to a neurologic disorder causing muscular imbalance contracture of the soft tissue structures.
Symptoms	General foot pain; pain in the ball of the foot; increase in incidence of overuse symptoms in the ankle, knee, hip, or back. The athlete may experience symptoms associated with peroneal tendinitis or plantar faciitis.
Signs	Clawed or hammer toes; tight plantar fascia; shortening of the achilles tendon; heavy calluses on the ball of the foot or heel; adduction of the forefoot; forefoot valgus in the frontal plane; heel varus in the frontal plane; excessive high medial longitudinal arch.
Special Tests	Not applicable
Referral/ Diagnostic Procedure	Not applicable
Classification of Injury	Not applicable

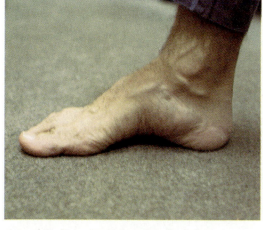 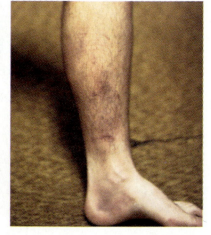

A and B, Pes cavus feet (high arch).

Medical Term	Pes planus foot
Common Term	Flat foot
Mechanisms	Congenital; poorly fitted shoes; muscle atrophy and loss of support; may follow rapid growth when muscle strength lags behind bony growth; obesity; excessive exercise; trauma to the support structures.
Symptoms	Pain in the medial longitudinal arch; loss of spring in step; stiffness; tiredness and tenderness in the medial longitudinal arch and heel; slight disability; possible low back pain and other areas of the lower extremity.
Signs	Everted position of the calcaneus; medial bulging of the navicular tuberosity; reduction in the height of the medial arch; first metatarsal bone usually dorsiflexed; tenderness in the medial arch; possible disability.
Special Tests	Not applicable
Referral/ Diagnostic Procedure	Not applicable
Classification of Injury	Not applicable

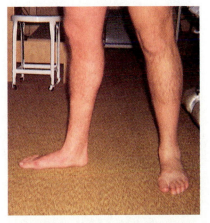

Pes planus foot (flat foot)

Medical Term	**Plantar fasciitis (strain)**
Common Term	Same as above
Mechanisms	Chronic overuse as in running; acute trauma; pes planus or pes cavus foot.
Symptoms	Pain on the plantar surface of the foot; sticking pain in the foot when taking the first steps in the morning.
Signs	Tenderness over the attachment of the plantar fascia on the medial tubercle of the calcaneus; pain that increases with dorsiflexion of the ankle.
Special Tests	Dorsiflexion of the ankle and extension of the toes may reproduce the pain.
Referral/ Diagnostic Procedure	Refer to an orthopedic surgeon if symptoms/signs persist. X– ray.
Classification of Injury	First-, second-, and third-degree. See Chapter 1 for classification of strain injury.

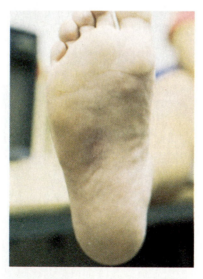

Ecchymosis on plantar surface
of the foot due to plantar
fasciitis (strain).

Medical Term	**Plantar neuroma/interdigital neuroma**
Common Term	Morton's neuroma
Mechanisms	A thickening of the plantar nerve at the point where the medial and lateral branches join and separate to pass to the adjacent sides of the third and fourth toes; the thick area pinches between the metatarsal heads; narrow shoes.
Symptoms	Intermittent, sharp pain in the lateral foot; sharp pain in the third and fourth toes; temporary loss of function.
Signs	Tenderness usually between the third and fourth metatarsal heads; palpation may reveal a small tender mass in the nerve.
Special Tests	Squeeze the metatarsal head together to reproduce the pain.
Referral/ Diagnostic Procedure	Refer to an orthopedic surgeon.
Classification of Injury	Not applicable

Medical Term	**Sesamoiditis**
Common Term	Same as above
Mechanisms	Indirect trauma caused by increased tension due to hyperextension of the great toe; roughening of the articular surface of the sesamoid bone.
Symptoms	Pain on weight bearing; tenderness over the sesamoid area on the plantar surface of the foot; possible loss of the ability to bear weight normally.
Signs	Abnormal gait; tenderness on palpation of the sesamoid bones; inflammation.
Special Tests	Not applicable
Referral/ Diagnostic Procedure	Refer to an orthopedic surgeon if symptoms/signs persist. X– ray.
Classification of Injury	Not applicable

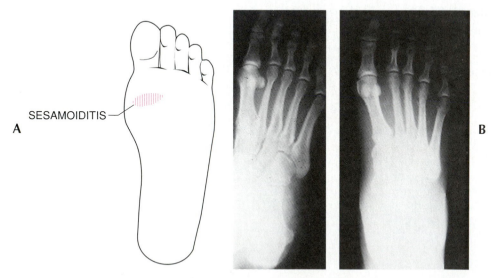

A, Area of pain for sesamoiditis. **B**, X-rays showing sesamoid bone.

Medical Term	**Anterior metatarsal arch sprain**
Common Term	Dropped metatarsal head
Mechanisms	Stress due to playing on a hard surface over a long period of time; weak ligaments or muscles; stretching of a ligament due to direct or indirect force applied to a joint.
Symptoms	Pain; a burning sensation; toe cramping; loss of function; tenderness.
Signs	Redness on the ball of the foot; callus formation on the plantar surface of the foot; pain produced by pressing down on the head of the affected metatarsal; point tenderness.
Special Tests	Pressing down from dorsal or plantar side on the head of the affected metatarsal produces pain.
Referral/ Diagnostic Procedure	Refer to an orthopedic surgeon if symptoms/signs persist.
Classification of Injury	First-, second-, and third-degree. See Chapter 1 for classification of sprain injury.

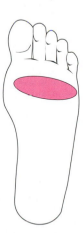

Area of pain for anterior metatarsal arch strain.

Medical Term	**Static arch sprain**
Common Term	Fallen arch
Mechanisms	Repeated episodes of overmotion; constant stress of superimposed weight on the arch of the foot; obesity.
Symptoms	Pain along the plantar calcaneonavicular ligament; tenderness; pain with weight bearing; loss of function.
Signs	Point tenderness over the plantar calcaneonavicular ligament; loss of function; swelling; hemorrhage; inflammation; inability to bear weight on the foot.
Special Tests	Not applicable
Referral/ Diagnostic Procedure	Refer to an orthopedic surgeon if symptoms/signs persist.
Classification of Injury	First-, second-, and third-degree. See Chapter 1 for classification of sprain injury.

Medical Term	**Traumatic arch sprain**
Common Term	Fallen arch
Mechanisms	Trauma; overuse; stretching of a ligament due to a direct or indirect force applied to a joint.
Symptoms	Pain and possible inability to weight bearing; pain on active and resistive movement; tenderness.
Signs	Point tenderness in the arch; swelling; hemorrhage; inability to weight bear.
Special Tests	Not applicable
Referral/ Diagnostic Procedure	Refer to an orthopedic surgeon if symptoms/signs persist.
Classification of Injury	First-, second-, and third-degree. See Chapter 1 for classification of sprain injury.

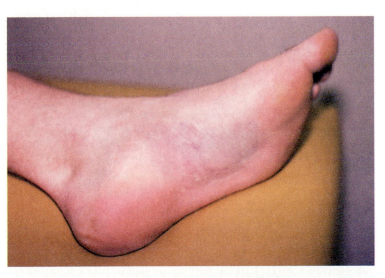

Swelling and ecchymosis of the anterior longitudinal arch.

Medical Term	**Great toe sprain**
Common Term	Turf toe
Mechanisms	Extreme dorsiflexion or plantar flexion of the metatarsophalangeal joint during push off; kicking a nonyielding object; overuse; stretching of a ligament due to a direct or indirect force applied to a joint.
Symptoms	Pain on active and resistive movement; pain on passive stress; loss of function; tenderness; abnormal gait.
Signs	Point tenderness over the first metatarsophalangeal joint; swelling; hemorrhage; possible deformity with third-degree injury; ecchymosis; possible instability with second- and third-degree injury; abnormal gait.
Special Tests	Assessment of range of motion and ligamentous stability.
Referral/ Diagnostic Procedure	Refer to an orthopedic surgeon. X–ray.
Classification of Injury	First-, second-, and third-degree. See Chapter 1 for classification of sprain injury.

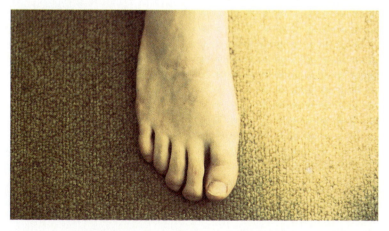

Swelling of the first metatarsophalangeal joint due to sprain.

Medical Term	**Tarsal tunnel syndrome**
Common Term	Same as above
Mechanisms	Entrapment of the posterior tibial nerve in the tunnel between the flexor retinaculum and the medial malleolus.
Symptoms	Paresthesia, mostly at night—hanging the foot out of the bed relieves the pain; pain in the medial longitudinal arch and in the ball of the foot.
Signs	Tenderness on palpation of the posterior tibial nerve.
Special Tests	Not applicable
Referral/ Diagnostic Procedure	Refer to an orthopedic surgeon.
Classification of Injury	Not applicable

Medical Term	**Unguis incarnates**
Common Term	Ingrown toe nail
Mechanisms	Improper footwear; improper cutting of the nail.
Symptoms	Pain; possible loss of activity in severe cases, redness.
Signs	Swelling; inflammation; improperly cut or deformed nail; possible infection; possible loss of function in severe cases.
Special Tests	Not applicable
Referral/ Diagnostic Procedure	Refer to a physician.
Classification of Injury	Not applicable

A 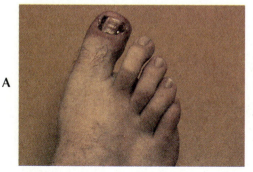 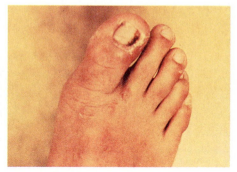 B

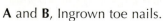

A and **B**, Ingrown toe nails.

Medical Term	*Verruca plantaris*
Common Term	Plantar wart
Mechanisms	Indirect cause of viral infection, abnormal friction or excessive weight bearing.
Symptoms	Localized pain with weight bearing; epidermal thickening; pain on direct pressure. The athlete complains of a pain that feels like walking on glass.
Signs	Wart growing inward. Warts may be singular or in clusters; usually found on the sole of the foot or areas of abnormal weight bearing. Pain on weight bearing.
Special Tests	Not applicable
Referral/ Diagnostic Procedure	Refer to a physician if symptoms/signs persist.
Classification of Injury	Not applicable

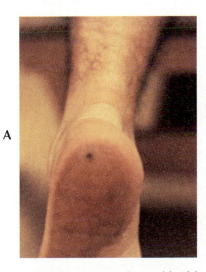
A
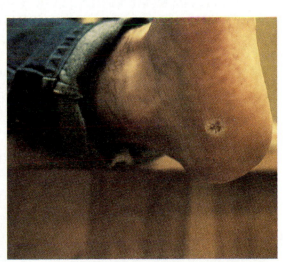
B

A, Plantar wart indicated by black area on plantar surface of heel. **B**, Plantar surface of heel following removal of wart.

■ TESTS FOR EVALUATION OF INJURIES TO THE ■ FOOT

(All tests should be performed bilaterally)

■ GENERAL ASSESSMENT TEST FOR RANGE OF MOTION AND STRENGTH FOR STRAIN, TENDINITIS, AND TENOSYNOVITIS

Active Movement

The athlete moves the body part through the range of motion actively, trying to reproduce the pain.

Passive Stretch

The athletic trainer performs a passive stretch of the involved muscle or tendon.

Resistive Movement

The athlete moves the body part through the range of motion while the athletic trainer applies resistance.

■ GENERAL ASSESSMENT TEST FOR RANGE OF MOTION AND LIGAMENTOUS STABILITY FOR A SPRAIN

Active Movement

The athlete moves the joint through the range of motion actively. The athletic trainer should be looking for any limitations in the range of motion.

Passive Movement

If the athlete cannot move the joint through the range of motion actively, then passive range of motion should be done to determine whether the range of motion is blocked due to the athlete's pain or because some object is blocking the joint.

Resistive Movement

The athlete moves the joint through the range of motion while the athletic trainer applies resistance.

Passive Stress

The athletic trainer applies stress to the joint to test the integrity of the ligamentous structures of the joint.

Skin Conditions

Chapter 19

Abrasion

Acne Vulgaris

Burn

Carbuncle

Actinic Dermatitis

Contact Dermatitis

Seborrheic Dermatitis

Folliculitis

Frostbite

Furunculosis

Hyperhidrosis

Impetigo

Intertrigo

Onychia

Paronychia

Pediculosis

Pityriasis Rosea

Prickly Heat

Psoriasis

Scabies

Sebaceous Cyst

Tinea Corporis

Tinea Cruris

Tinea Pedis

Urticaria

Verruca Vulgaris

Medical Term	**Abrasion**
Common Term	Strawberry
Mechanisms	Scraping skin against a rough surface.
Symptoms	Pain.
Signs	Skin that is worn away or rubbed off, oozing and bleeding.
Special Tests	Not applicable
Referral/ Diagnostic Procedure	Refer to a physician if symptoms/signs persist.
Classification of Injury	Not applicable

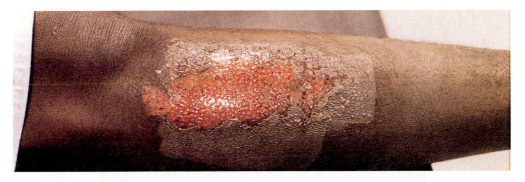

Abrasion.

Medical Term	**Acne vulgaris**
Common Term	Acne
Mechanisms	Inflammation of sebaceous glands and hair follicles. Most common during puberty.
Symptoms	Possible pain and itching.
Signs	Blackheads; cysts; pustules.
Special Tests	Not applicable
Referral/ Diagnostic Procedure	Refer to a dermatologist.
Classification of Injury	Not applicable

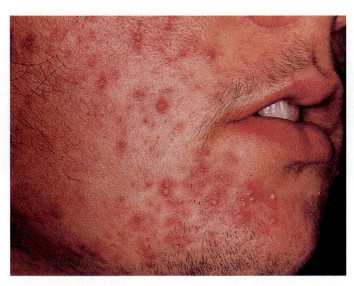

Many pustules are present, and several have become confluent on the chin area.

Medical Term	Burn
Common Term	Same as above
Mechanisms	Excessive exposure to thermal, chemical, or electrical agents.
Symptoms	Shock; pain.
Signs	Blisters, charring, redness.
Special Tests	Not applicable
Referral/ Diagnostic Procedure	Refer to a dermatologist.
Classification of Injury	Partial-thickness (first-degree and second-degree) burns damage the top layer of skin and can damage the epidermis and upper layers of the dermis; full-thickness (third-degree) burns destroy both the epidermis and dermis.

Medical Term	Carbuncle
Common Term	Boil
Mechanisms	Bacterial infection.
Symptoms	Painful node occurring most often on the back of the neck.
Signs	Reddish skin; early dark, red, hard area changing to a lesion with yellow–red pus; inflammation.
Special Tests	Not applicable
Referral/ Diagnostic Procedure	Refer to a dermatologist. Possible internal infection that can spread to other athletes.
Classification of Injury	Not applicable

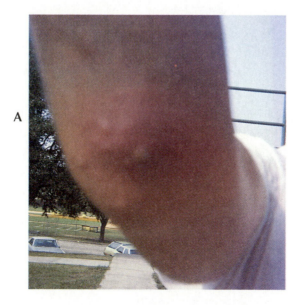

A

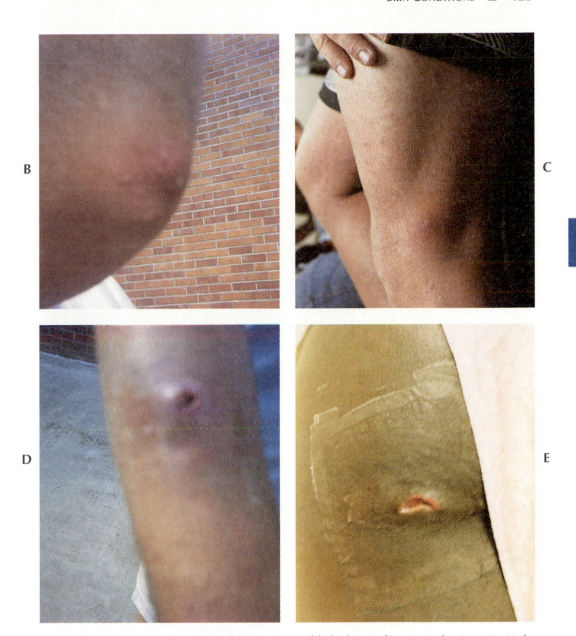

A and B, Beginning of area of infection. C, Reddish skin indicating infection. D, Hole after removal of core. E, Boil after being lanced.

Medical Term	**Actinic dermatitis**
Common Term	Sunburn
Mechanisms	Overexposure to the sun.
Symptoms	Itching, possible shock.
Signs	Swelling, blistering, erythema.
Special Tests	Not applicable
Referral/ Diagnostic Procedure	Refer to a dermatologist if symptoms/signs persist.
Classification of Injury	Not applicable

Medical Term	**Contact dermatitis**
Common Term	Allergic reaction.
Mechanisms	Exposure to an irritating substance.
Symptoms	Itching.
Signs	Redness of the skin, swelling, vesicles that may ooze and form a crust.
Special Tests	Not applicable
Referral/ Diagnostic Procedure	Refer to a dermatologist.
Classification of Injury	Not applicable

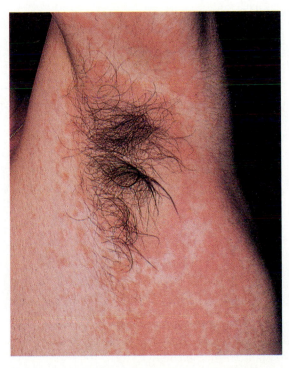

Allergic contact dermatitis to a spray deodorant.

Medical Term	**Seborrheic dermatitis**
Common Term	Same as above
Mechanisms	Not applicable
Symptoms	None
Signs	Round, irregular lesion with yellowish scales on the scalp that can spread to the forehead.
Special Tests	Not applicable
Referral/ Diagnostic Procedure	Refer to a dermatologist.
Classification of Injury	Not applicable

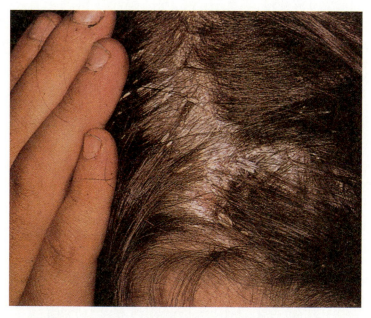

Seborrheic dermatitis (tinea amiantacea). The scalp contains dense patches of scale. Large plates of yellow-white scale firmly adhere to the hair shafts.

Medical Term	Folliculitis
Common Term	Infected hair.
Mechanisms	Infection of a hair follicle.
Symptoms	Possible pain.
Signs	Inflammation, pustule that may develop a crust.
Special Tests	Not applicable
Referral/ Diagnostic Procedure	Refer to a dermatologist.
Classification of Injury	Not applicable

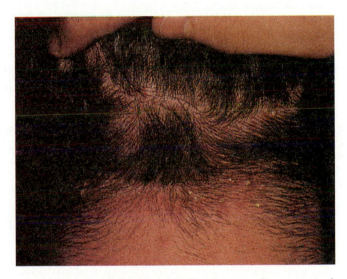

Staphylococcal folliculitis. Follicular pustules appeared after the patient's lower extremity had been occluded with a topical steroid and a plastic dressing for 24 hours. Gram-negative organisms may also flourish after long periods of plastic occlusion.

Medical Term	Frostbite
Common Term	Same as above
Mechanisms	Freezing of superficial or deep tissue.
Symptoms	Itching and numbness in mild cases; paresthesia and stiffness in moderate cases; numbness and tissue death in severe cases.
Signs	The skin in the injured area is cold, hard, white, and anesthetic. Upon rewarming the area stings, burns, turns blotchy red, and will swell. Possible blistering in moderate cases; possible tissue death in severe cases, with gangrene due to the tissue death.
Special Tests	Not applicable
Referral/ Diagnostic Procedure	Refer for immediate medical attention.
Classification of Injury	First-degree superficial, second-degree superficial, second-degree deep, and third-degree deep frostbite.

A 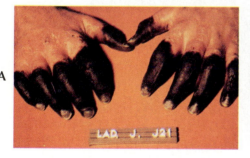 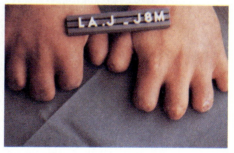 B

A, Third-degree deep frostbite. **B**, Same patient after 8 months.

Medical Term	**Furunculosis**
Common Term	Boil
Mechanisms	Bacterial infection occurring from irritation of hair follicles or sebaceous gland.
Symptoms	Pain in the area of infection.
Signs	Redness; presence of a pustule that is hard from internal pressure and tender to palpation.
Special Tests	Not applicable
Referral/ Diagnostic Procedure	Refer to a dermatologist.
Classification of Injury	Not applicable

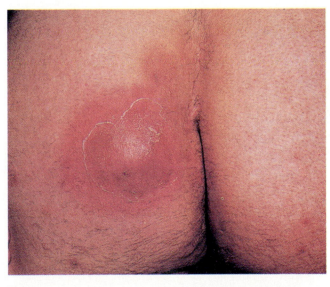

Enlarged swollen mass with purulent material beginning to exude from several points on the surface.

Medical Term	**Hyperhidrosis**
Common Term	Sweating
Mechanisms	Overactivity of sweat glands, caused by disease or stimulant use.
Symptoms	See signs.
Signs	Excessive sweating of the hands and feet.
Special Tests	Not applicable
Referral/ Diagnostic Procedure	Refer to a physician.
Classification of Injury	Not applicable

Medical Term	Impetigo
Common Term	Same as above
Mechanisms	Bacterial infection, which is common in wrestlers. Occurs most around the mouth and nostrils.
Symptoms	Itching, soreness.
Signs	Lesions vary from pea-sized vesicopustule to large, bizarre, circular lesions with yellowish crustation on the skin.
Special Tests	Not applicable
Referral/ Diagnostic Procedure	Refer to a dermatologist.
Classification of Injury	Not applicable

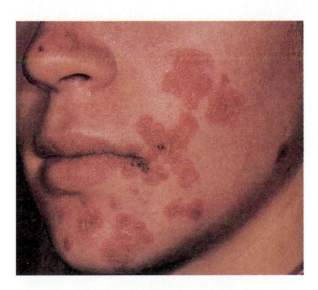

Lesions are present in all stages of development. Bullae rupture, exposing a lesion with an eroded surface and peripheral scale.

Medical Term	Intertrigo
Common Term	Chafing
Mechanisms	Friction and softening in the folds of the skin from heat and moisture.
Symptoms	Pain and chafing.
Signs	Erythema; possibly an oozing wound.
Special Tests	Not applicable
Referral/ Diagnostic Procedure	Refer to a dermatologist.
Classification of Injury	Not applicable

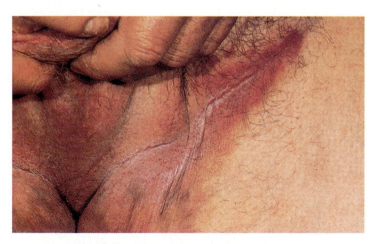

A tender red plaque with a moist macerated surface extends to an equal extent onto the scrotum and thigh.

Medical Term	Onychia
Common Term	Nail bed infection
Mechanisms	Fungal infection.
Symptoms	Pain.
Signs	Inflammation at nailbed; possible loss of nail; white or yellow discoloration of subungual area.
Special Tests	Not applicable
Referral/ Diagnostic Procedure	Refer to a physician.
Classification of Injury	Not applicable

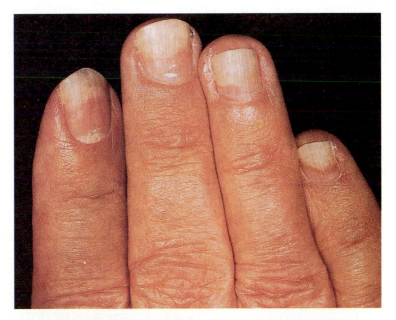

Separation of the nail plate starts at the distal groove. Minor trauma to long fingernails is the most common cause.

Medical Term	Paronychia
Common Term	Same as above
Mechanisms	Bacterial or fungal infection. Trauma to the nail bed or end of the finger.
Symptoms	Pain around the nail bed.
Signs	Redness, swelling, and possibly pus formation seen near a fingernail or toenail.
Special Tests	Not applicable
Referral/ Diagnostic Procedure	Refer to a physician.
Classification of Injury	Not applicable

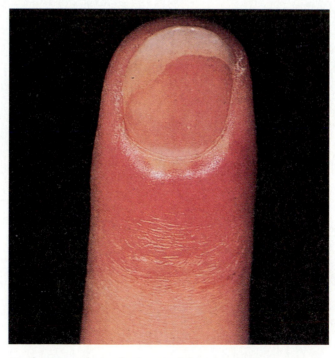

Erythema and purulent material occur at the proximal nail fold.

Medical Term	Pediculosis
Common Term	Body lice
Mechanisms	Infestation of lice.
Symptoms	Itching and scratching.
Signs	May lead to secondary infection and formation of pustules and crusts. The hair may become matted, and small, ovoid, grayish white nits may be visible fixed to hair shafts.
Special Tests	Not applicable
Referral/ Diagnostic Procedure	Refer to a dermatologist.
Classification of Injury	Not applicable

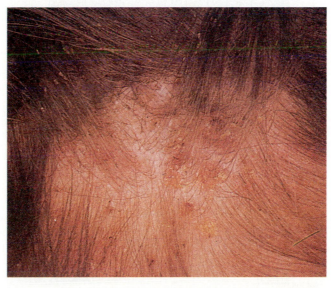

Human lice can spread from the pubic area to involve the axillae.

Medical Term	**Pityriasis rosea**
Common Term	Same as above
Mechanisms	Unknown infection.
Symptoms	See signs.
Signs	Redness and branny scales with an oval raised border, usually on the trunk of the body. It resembles superficial ringworm.
Special Tests	Not applicable
Referral/ Diagnostic Procedure	Refer to a dermatologist.
Classification of Injury	Not applicable

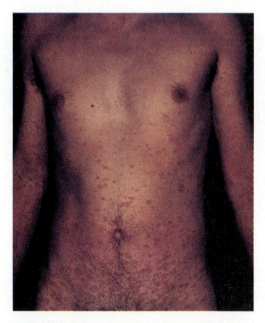

Pityriasis rosea. Both small oval plaques and multiple small papules are present. Occasionally the eruption will consist only of small papules.

Medical Term	**Prickly heat**
Common Term	Same as above
Mechanisms	Common temperature reaction; a result of exposure to heat and moisture.
Symptoms	Itching.
Signs	Pustules and burning vesicles.
Special Tests	Not applicable
Referral/ Diagnostic Procedure	Refer to a dermatologist.
Classification of Injury	Not applicable

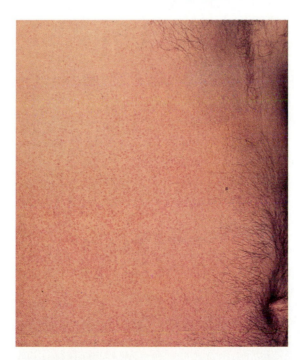

A diffuse eruption of tiny papules and vesicles occurs after exertion or overheating.

Medical Term	Psoriasis
Common Term	Same as above
Mechanisms	Unknown; may be a result of increased epidermal cell proliferation.
Symptoms	Discomfort.
Signs	Flat-topped papules covered with thin, grayish-white scales; under dry scales are red bleeding points; lesions are sharply demarcated. This is a chronic condition, although it comes and goes.
Special Tests	Not applicable
Referral/ Diagnostic Procedure	Refer to a dermatologist.
Classification of Injury	Not applicable

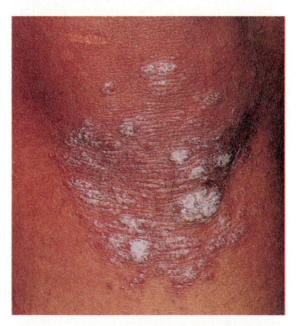

Pustular psoriasis of the digits. The eruption has remained localized in this one finger for years.

Medical Term	Scabies
Common Term	Seven-year itch
Mechanisms	Parasitic skin infection caused by the mite *Sarcoptes scabiei*.
Symptoms	Nocturnal itching.
Signs	Parasite burrows, approximately ¼ to ½ inch (0.5 to 1.0 cm) below the skin surface, between fingers and toes, wrists, axillae, nipples, inside of thighs, beltline, and buttocks.
Special Tests	Not applicable
Referral/ Diagnostic Procedure	Refer to a dermatologist.
Classification of Injury	Not applicable

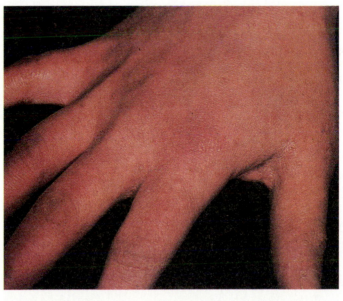

Scabies. Tiny vesicles and papules in the finger webs and back of the hand.

Medical Term	**Sebaceous cyst**
Common Term	Wens
Mechanisms	Slow-growing, benign cystic tumor.
Symptoms	Discomfort if infected.
Signs	Small sac with sebaceous matter, movable and not sore.
Special Tests	Not applicable
Referral/ Diagnostic Procedure	Refer to a dermatologist.
Classification of Injury	Not applicable

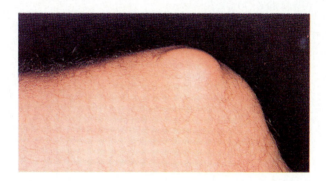

A sebaceous cyst can occur in uncommon places.

Medical Term	**Tinea corporis**
Common Term	Ringworm
Mechanisms	Dermatophyte infection.
Symptoms	Itching.
Signs	Slightly elevated scaly patches; a circular pattern of vesicular areas.
Special Tests	Not applicable
Referral/ Diagnostic Procedure	Refer to a dermatologist.
Classification of Injury	Not applicable

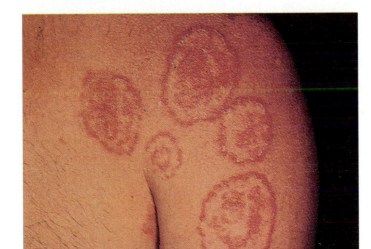

Tinea corposis. A classic presentation with an advancing red scaly border. The reason for the designation "ringworm" is obvious.

Medical Term	**Tinea cruris**
Common Term	Jock itch
Mechanisms	Fungal infection
Symptoms	Itching, pain, and discomfort associated with infection.
Signs	Redness.
Special Tests	Not applicable
Referral/ Diagnostic Procedure	Refer to a dermatologist if symptoms/signs persist.
Classification of Injury	Not applicable

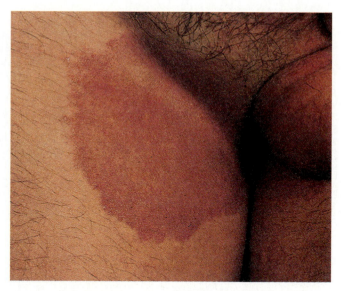

Tinea cruris. A half-moon–shaped plaque has a well-defined scaling border.

Medical Term	**Tinea pedis**
Common Term	Athlete's foot
Mechanisms	Fungal infection.
Symptoms	Itching.
Signs	Inflammation of tissue; possible infection; cracking of skin; rash; blisters.
Special Tests	Not applicable
Referral/ Diagnostic Procedure	Refer to a dermatologist if symptoms/signs persist.
Classification of Injury	Not applicable

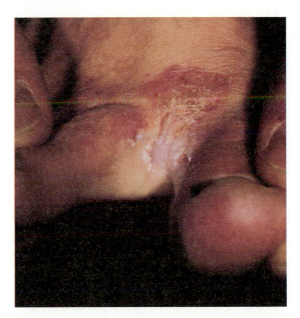

Tinea pedis (toe web infection). The toe web space contains macerated scale. Inflammation has extended from the web area onto the dorsum of the foot.

Medical Term	**Urticaria**
Common Term	Hives
Mechanisms	Allergic reaction to food, substance, insect bite, heat, pollen, or drugs.
Symptoms	Intense itching.
Signs	Rash.
Special Tests	Not applicable
Referral/ Diagnostic Procedure	Refer to a dermatologist.
Classification of Injury	Not applicable

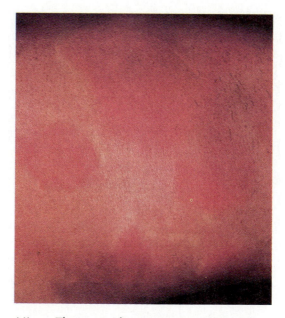

Hives. The most characteristic presentation is uniformly red edematous plaques surrounded by a faint white halo. These superficial lesions occur from transcudation of fluid into the dermis.

Medical Term	**Verruca vulgaris**
Common Term	Common wart
Mechanisms	Viral infection.
Symptoms	See signs.
Signs	Small, round, elevated lesion with rough, dry surface, located on the hand or foot. The wart may contain markings resembling small black seeds.
Special Tests	Not applicable
Referral/ Diagnostic Procedure	Refer to a dermatologist if symptoms/signs persist.
Classification of Injury	Not applicable

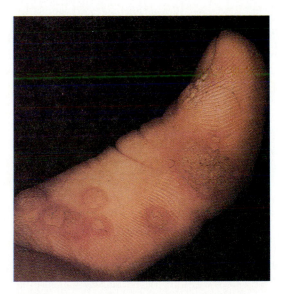

Common warts with thrombosed vessels
(black dots) on the surface.

GENERAL MEDICAL CONDITIONS

Chapter 20

Amenorrhea
Anemia
Appendicitis
Asthma
Autoimmune Deficiency Syndrome
  (AIDS)/Human Immunodeficiency
  Virus (HIV)
Bronchitis
Cellulitis
Chlamydia
Coccidiomycosis
Colitis
Condyloma Acuminata
Constipation
Diabetes Mellitus
Diarrhea
Dysmenorrhea
Epilepsy/Seizure Disorder
Gastritis
Gastroenteritis
Gonorrhea
Gynecomastia
Hemorrhoids
Herpes Simplex Virus, Type I
Herpes Simplex Virus, Type II
Traumatic Tunica Vaginalis
  Hydrocele

Hypertension
Hyperventilation
Hypothermia
Indigestion
Influenza
Insect Bites and Stings
Laryngitis
Mononucleosis
Mumps
Pancreatitis
Pharyngitis
Pneumonia
Rhinitis
Rhinitis, Allergic
Rubella
Rubeola
Sickle Cell Anemia
Sinusitis
Tinea Versicolor
Tetanus
Tonsillitis
Upper Respiratory Infection
Urethritis
Urinary Tract Infection
Vaginitis
Varicella
Viral Hepatitis

Medical Term	**Amenorrhea**
Common Term	Same as above
Mechanisms	Hard physical training; low body fat; medical abnormalities in female athletes such as crash dieting, obesity, emotional stress, or illness.
Symptoms	None
Signs	Absence of menses.
Special Tests	Not applicable
Referral/ Diagnostic Procedure	Refer the athlete to a physician.
Classification of Injury	Not applicable

Medical Term	Anemia
Common Term	Same as above
Mechanisms	Low level of normal hemoglobin; destruction of red blood cells; impaired red blood cell production; excessive blood loss.
Symptoms	Low exercise tolerance; easy fatigue; dizziness on rising from recumbent or sitting position, weakness, drowsiness, tachycardia.
Signs	Elevated resting pulse rate; pale skin and mucous membranes.
Special Tests	Not applicable
Referral/ Diagnostic Procedure	Refer to physician. Hemoglobin/hematocrit counts.
Classification of Injury	Not applicable

Medical Term	**Appendicitis**
Common Term	Same as above
Mechanisms	Inflammation and possible infection of the appendix.
Symptoms	Nausea; pain in the right lower quadrant of the abdomen; anorexia.
Signs	Vomiting; fever; tenderness that is usually in the right lower quadrant of the abdomen, but the location may be variable, especially early in the course. Acute abdomen signs with perforation of the appendix.
Special Tests	Positive rebound test. (See p. 257 for description of test.)
Referral/ Diagnostic Procedure	Refer to general surgeon. CBC.
Classification of Injury	Not applicable

Medical Term	Asthma
Common Term	Same as above
Mechanisms	Widespread airway narrowing and obstruction that is reversible either spontaneously or as a result of medication. Asthma is felt to be allergy-based.
Symptoms	Dyspnea; "air hunger;" shortness of breath; wheezing; cough.
Signs	Wheezing, with expiratory phase of respiration longer than inspiratory; tachycardia; tachypnea; and diaphoresis. Some patients may develop attacks of asthma only after or during exercise; this is called "exercise-induced asthma."
Special Tests	Not applicable
Referral/ Diagnostic Procedure	Refer to a physician with pulmonary expertise. Pulmonary function studies; chest x-ray is sometimes helpful.
Classification of Injury	Not applicable

Medical Term	Autoimmune deficiency syndrome/human immunodeficiency virus
Common Term	AIDS
Mechanisms	The attack of white blood cells, in particular lymphocytes, by HIV. After a variable number of years, secondary infections such as pneumonia and yeast slowly lead to deterioration and, ultimately, death.
Symptoms	None for HIV infection. Numerous symptoms, such as cough, malaise, headache, and skin rashes, can be seen with the secondary infection phase.
Signs	None for HIV infection. Fever; abnormal lung sounds; noticeably ill appearance; and a number of other signs, depending on the nature of the secondary infection.
Special Tests	Not applicable
Referral/ Diagnostic Procedure	Refer to a physician.
Classification of Injury	Not applicable

Medical Term	Bronchitis
Common Term	Same as above
Mechanisms	Viral or bacterial infection of bronchial tubes. Edema and secretions are usually present.
Symptoms	Cough that is productive of yellow-green colored sputum; chills; possibly chest pain; sometimes shortness of breath.
Signs	Fever; sometimes audible breath sounds; lethargy; cough.
Special Tests	Not applicable
Referral/ Diagnostic Procedure	Refer to physician with pulmonary expertise.
Classification of Injury	Not applicable

Medical Term	Cellulitis
Common Term	Same as above
Mechanisms	Inflammation and swelling of skin and underlying tissues; secondary to bacterial infection.
Symptoms	Swelling and tenderness in a localized area of the skin.
Signs	Erythema; edema; tenderness in a localized area of the body.
Special Tests	Not applicable
Referral/ Diagnostic Procedure	Refer to a physician. Take the patient's temperature; culture site, if open; obtain CBC.
Classification of Injury	Not applicable

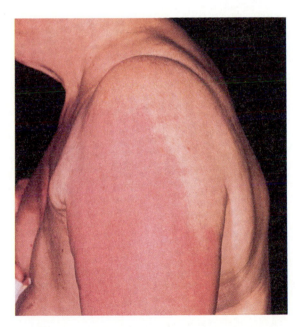

Cellulitis.

Medical Term	Chlamydia
Common Term	Venereal disease
Mechanisms	Spread by sexual contact.
Symptoms	Possible dysuria; possible dyspareunia in females; pelvic pain in advanced cases in females.
Signs	Colored vaginal or penile discharge; possible pain with manipulation of cervix.
Special Tests	Not applicable
Referral/ Diagnostic Procedure	Refer to physician for chlamydia screen; CBC in more severe cases.
Classification of Injury	Not applicable

Medical Term	Coccidiomycosis
Common Term	Same as above
Mechanisms	Infection with *Coccidioides immitis*, a fungus which occurs in the primary form as an acute, benign, self–limiting respiratory disease.
Symptoms	Patient may be asymptomatic, or may present with a cough, chest pain, chills, a sore throat, and hemoptysis.
Signs	Occasional scattered rales on lung exam. May have fever.
Special Tests	Not applicable
Referral/ Diagnostic Procedure	Refer to a physician with pulmonary expertise for sputum samples for the fungus. This disease is endemic in the southwest United States.
Classification of Injury	Not applicable

Medical Term	Colitis
Common Term	Same as above
Mechanisms	Inflammation of large bowel, secondary to infection or chronic bowel disease such as ulcerative colitis or Crohn's disease.
Symptoms	Diarrhea, often bloody, with mucus present. Episodes of lower abdominal pain with increased flatus may also be present.
Signs	Noticeably ill appearance. Abdomen may be tender to palpation, and fever may be present.
Special Tests	Not applicable
Referral/ Diagnostic Procedure	Refer to a physician. Hemoccult stool; stool culture; and stool for parasites.
Classification of Injury	Not applicable

Medical Term	**Condyloma acuminata**
Common Term	Venereal warts
Mechanisms	Human papilloma virus.
Symptoms	None.
Signs	Lesions ranging in appearance from warty to moist fungoid. May be single or multiple, in a variety of sizes.
Special Tests	None
Referral/ Diagnostic Procedure	Refer to a physician.
Classification of Injury	Not applicable

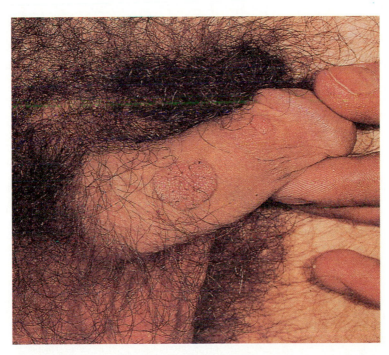

Condyloma acuminata on the shaft of the penis.

Medical Term	Constipation
Common Term	Same as above
Mechanisms	Decreased motility (spontaneous movement) of large bowel and decreased fluid content of feces.
Symptoms	Hard stool with straining during bowel movements; bloated feeling with decreased appetite; headache.
Signs	Diagnosis is made from patient's history. It should be noted that not frequency but hardness of bowel movements is the key.
Special Tests	None
Referral/ Diagnostic Procedure	Refer to a physician if symptoms/signs persist. Hemoccult of stool is sometimes done.
Classification of Injury	Not applicable

Medical Term	**Diabetes mellitus (Non–insulin-dependent diabetes mellitus [NIDDM], insulin-dependent diabetes mellitus [IDDM])**
Common Term	Sugar diabetes
Mechanisms	A disorder of glucose metabolism, involving abnormal insulin production by the pancreas and/or inability of the body to properly utilize glucose at the cellular level.
Symptoms	Polyuria; polydipsia (excessive thirst); sometimes lethargy; weight gain or loss; in severe cases coma, leading to death if not treated immediately.
Signs	Usually none until the patient begins to approach a seriously high level, leading to lethargy and coma.
Special Tests	Not applicable
Referral/ Diagnostic Procedure	Refer to a physician. Blood glucose; potassium.
Classification of Injury	Not applicable

Medical Term	Diarrhea
Common Term	Same as above
Mechanisms	Loss of ability of the large bowel to absorb fluids, secondary to damage to the cell lining of the bowel. This damage has many etiologies, including viral, bacterial, and protozoal, among others.
Symptoms	Loose, watery bowel movements. Diarrhea is defined by the consistency of the stool, not by the frequency.
Signs	Fever may be present with infectious diarrhea; blood may be noted in the stool.
Special Tests	Not applicable
Referral/ Diagnostic Procedure	Refer to a physician if symptoms/signs persist. Stool hemocult and stool cultures are sometimes done. Studies for ova, cysts, and parasites (OCP) may be ordered.
Classification of Injury	Not applicable

Medical Term	**Dysmenorrhea**
Common Term	Same as above
Mechanisms	Lack of proper blood flow to pelvic organs; hormonal imbalance in female athletes.
Symptoms	Painful menstruation; cramps; headache; lower abdominal pain; changing emotional state; nausea.
Signs	Abdominal tenderness during menstruation.
Special Tests	Not applicable
Referral/ Diagnostic Procedure	Refer to a physician.
Classification of Injury	Not applicable

Medical Term	**Epilepsy/seizure disorder**
Common Term	Seizures
Mechanisms	Disorder of the brain that causes intermittent episodes of symptoms; these range from brief breaks in the consciousness to total body tonic–clonic seizures that lead to unconsciousness.
Symptoms	May have aura (change in vision or smell) before seizure.
Signs	The obvious tonic–clonic seizure is easily diagnosed, but more subtle seizures include brief breaks in consciousness that do not involve totally losing consciousness.
Special Tests	Not applicable
Referral/ Diagnostic Procedure	Refer to neurologist if seizure occurs. Electroencephalogram (EEG) and CT head to rule out tumor in brain.
Classification of Injury	Not applicable

Medical Term	Gastritis
Common Term	Stomachache; heartburn
Mechanisms	Inflammation of the lining of the stomach due to increased acid; certain medications (i.e., aspirin); certain infectious agents.
Symptoms	Burning ache at the epigastric area of the abdomen.
Signs	Tenderness to palpation at the epigastric area.
Special Tests	Not applicable
Referral/ Diagnostic Procedure	Refer to a gastroenterologist.
Classification of Injury	Not applicable

Medical Term	Gastroenteritis
Common Term	Stomach flu/food poisoning
Mechanisms	Usually viral, but sometimes bacterial, infection of the gastrointestinal tract.
Symptoms	Nausea; vomiting; diarrhea; anorexia; sometimes abdominal gas cramping.
Signs	Fever and vomiting. Abdomen may be soft but diffusely tender, and skin and mucous membranes may be dry, if dehydrated.
Special Tests	Not applicable
Referral/ Diagnostic Procedure	Refer to a gastroenterologist. CBC, electrolytes, and stool cultures in severe cases.
Classification of Injury	Not applicable

Medical Term	**Gonorrhea**
Common Term	Clap, venereal disease
Mechanisms	Bacterial infection spread by sexual contact.
Symptoms	Dysuria; dyspareunia in females; pelvic pain in advanced cases in females.
Signs	Colored vaginal or penile discharge; possible pain with manipulation of cervix.
Special Tests	Not applicable
Referral/ Diagnostic Procedure	Refer to a physician for gonorrhea (G/C) culture; CBC in more severe cases.
Classification of Injury	Not applicable

Medical Term	Gynecomastia
Common Term	Same as above
Mechanisms	Discoid enlargement of breast tissue beneath the areola. Usually bilateral in pubescent boys and unilateral in men over 50. It is usually physiologic, and tends to resolve within 6 to 12 months. Rare cases include pituitary and testicular tumors. Use of anabolic steroids can be a factor.
Symptoms	Nontender enlargement of breast tissue in a male.
Signs	See symptoms.
Special Tests	Not applicable
Referral/ Diagnostic Procedure	Refer to a physician.
Classification of Injury	Not applicable

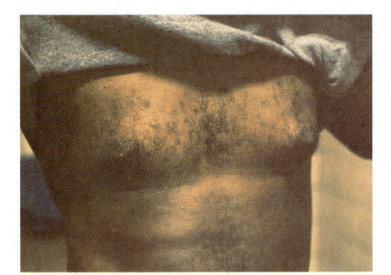

Enlargement of breast tissue indicating gynecomastia.

Medical Term	Hemorrhoids
Common Term	Piles
Mechanisms	Constipation; straining.
Symptoms	Pain; itching.
Signs	Swelling near sphincter of anus; bleeding.
Special Tests	Not applicable
Referral/ Diagnostic Procedure	Refer to a physician if symptoms/signs persist.
Classification of Injury	Not applicable

Medical Term	**Herpes simplex virus, type I**
Common Term	Cold sores, fever blisters
Mechanisms	Herpes virus infection.
Symptoms	Painful blisters on lips, in mouth, and sometimes in nose.
Signs	Clear vesicles on above-described areas. Vesicles are usually recurrent and may last from 1 to 2 weeks.
Special Tests	Not applicable
Referral/ Diagnostic Procedure	Refer to a physician. May culture lesions or draw blood antibody titer.
Classification of Injury	Not applicable

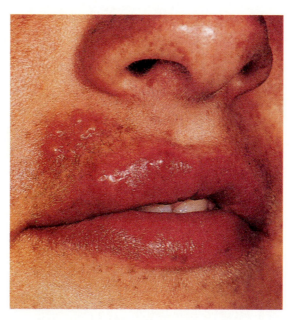

Fever blisters.

Medical Term	**Herpes simplex virus, type II**
Common Term	Genital herpes
Mechanisms	Herpes virus infection, with first outbreak usually 7 to 10 days after exposure.
Symptoms	Painful blisters located on or near genital organs. Burning lancinating pain may be present before blisters appear. Dysuria can be present with urethral involvement. The first attack is the most painful.
Signs	Single or multiple clear vesicles on red background; often have inguinal lymphadenopathy.
Special Tests	Not applicable
Referral/ Diagnostic Procedure	Refer to a physician. May culture lesions or draw blood antibody titer.
Classification of Injury	Not applicable

Medical Term	**Traumatic tunica vaginalis hydrocele**
Common Term	Fluid in scrotum
Mechanisms	Direct contact.
Symptoms	Pain; nausea; weakness.
Signs	Swelling.
Special Tests	Not applicable
Referral/ Diagnostic Procedure	Refer to a physician.
Classification of Injury	Not applicable

Medical Term	Hypertension
Common Term	High blood pressure
Mechanisms	An increased hydrostatic pressure of the blood brought on by increased peripheral resistance and/or increased cardiac output.
Symptoms	Usually none in mild to moderate hypertension. In severe hypertension, the patient may have headache, experience change in consciousness such as confusion, or lose equilibrium.
Signs	Increased systolic and/or diastolic pressure, with neurologic changes in severe cases.
Special Tests	Not applicable
Referral/ Diagnostic Procedure	Refer to a physician.
Classification of Injury	Not applicable

Medical Term	Hyperventilation
Common Term	Same as above
Mechanisms	Respiratory alkalosis due to an increased respiratory rate, causing an inadequate amount of carbon dioxide in the body. This deficit in turn leads to anxiety, apprehension, and neurologic changes such as numbness and tingling of the mouth and extremities.
Symptoms	See mechanisms.
Signs	Increased respiratory rate; anxiety.
Special Tests	Not applicable
Referral/ Diagnostic Procedure	Refer to physician if debilitating or if symptoms/signs persist.
Classification of Injury	Not applicable

Medical Term	**Hypothermia**
Common Term	Same as above
Mechanisms	Loss of body heat, leading to neurologic and electrical changes in the body and heart.
Symptoms	A spectrum of symptoms; can begin with shivering and can proceed to sluggish thinking, eventual loss of shivering, coma, failure of cardiac and respiratory centers, and finally death.
Signs	See symptoms. Loss of shivering is a sign of deepening hypothermia.
Special Tests	Not applicable
Referral/ Diagnostic Procedure	Refer to physician.
Classification of Injury	Not applicable

Medical Term	Indigestion
Common Term	Heartburn; stomachache; gas pains
Mechanisms	Increased amount of gas produced during digestion, along with increased acid output that leads to irritation of the esophagus, stomach, and intestine.
Symptoms	Substernal burning (heartburn); epigastric discomfort; bloating; intermittent sharp pain (gas pain) in the abdomen.
Signs	Diffuse abdominal tenderness without rigidity. Bowel sounds may be increased.
Special Tests	Not applicable
Referral/ Diagnostic Procedure	Refer to a physician if symptoms/signs persist.
Classification of Injury	Not applicable

Medical Term	**Influenza**
Common Term	Flu
Mechanisms	Influenza virus attacks upper airways, which leads to inflammation of these tissues and spread of the virus throughout the body via the bloodstream.
Symptoms	Headache; cough; chills; sinus stuffiness; myalgia (muscle pain); sore throat; malaise; fatigue.
Signs	Fever; postnasal drip; obvious illness.
Special Tests	Not applicable
Referral/ Diagnostic Procedure	Refer to a physician.
Classification of Injury	Not applicable

Medical Term	**Insect bites and stings**
Common Term	Same as above
Mechanisms	Body's immune reaction to toxin released by bites and stings.
Symptoms	Pain and swelling at the site. More extreme reactions may present with itching, swelling, and redness anywhere on the body. Shortness of breath and anxiety are found in respiratory involvement.
Signs	Swelling and redness at the site, with generalized urticarial-type rash. Wheezing may be noted in lung or pharyngeal involvement.
Special Tests	Not applicable
Referral/ Diagnostic Procedure	Refer to a physician if symptoms/signs persist.
Classification of Injury	Not applicable

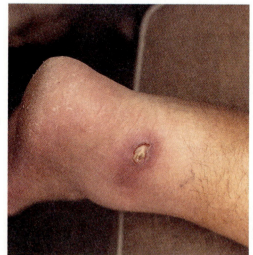 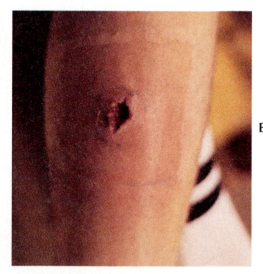

A, Insect bite. **B**, Spider bite.

Medical Term	**Laryngitis**
Common Term	Same as above
Mechanisms	Viral infection causing edema of the vocal cords, leading to loss of vocal ability.
Symptoms	Can include sore throat, runny nose, and postnasal drip.
Signs	Partial or complete loss of voice; possible cervical lymphadenopathy.
Special Tests	Not applicable
Referral/ Diagnostic Procedure	Refer to a physician.
Classification of Injury	Not applicable

Medical Term	Mononucleosis
Common Term	Mono
Mechanisms	Infection caused by Epstein-Barr virus, which primarily infects the lymphatic system.
Symptoms	Headache; malaise; sore throat; easy fatiguability.
Signs	Fever; exudative pharyngitis; anterior and posterior cervical adenopathy; sometimes general lympha-denopathy; spleen may be enlarged.
Special Tests	Not applicable
Referral/ Diagnostic Procedure	Refer to a physician. Blood test for mononucleosis. Sometimes CBC.
Classification of Injury	Not applicable

Medical Term	**Mumps**
Common Term	Same as above
Mechanisms	Infection of the parotid glands with the mumps virus. Up to 20% of males may develop orchitis, which, if bilateral, could lead to sterility.
Symptoms	Unilateral or bilateral swelling of the parotid glands; chills; headache; pain below the ears.
Signs	Swollen parotid glands; fever 101° to 102° F (38° to 39° C); painful jaw movement. If one cannot palpate the angle of the mandible, then mumps should be suspected.
Special Tests	Not applicable
Referral/ Diagnostic Procedure	Refer to a physician.
Classification of Injury	Not applicable

Medical Term	Pancreatitis
Common Term	Same as above
Mechanisms	Inflammation of the pancreas, usually caused by gallstones, alcohol use, or drug use.
Symptoms	Nausea; vomiting; anorexia, with abdominal pain; constipation.
Signs	Noticeably ill appearance; rapid pulse; clammy skin; fever; upper abdominal pain; possible jaundice; possible abdominal rigidity.
Special Tests	Not applicable
Referral/ Diagnostic Procedure	Refer to a gastroenterologist. Serum amylase.
Classification of Injury	Not applicable

Medical Term	Pharyngitis
Common Term	Throat infection
Mechanisms	Viral or bacterial infection of pharynx.
Symptoms	Sore throat; chills; lethargy; possibly headache.
Signs	Throat reddened, with or without pus; anterior cervical lymphadenopathy.
Special Tests	Not applicable
Referral/ Diagnostic Procedure	Refer to a physician. Strep screen and mononucleosis screen.
Classification of Injury	Not applicable

Medical Term	Pneumonia
Common Term	Same as above
Mechanisms	Viral or bacterial infection in lungs causing consolidation of fluids and white blood cells in one or more lobes of the lungs.
Symptoms	Cough with or without production of sputum; chills; shortness of breath; fatigue; anorexia; pain in the chest.
Signs	Fever; respiratory distress; elevated respiratory rate; elevated pulse; bronchial breath sounds on auscultation; dullness to percussion; chills.
Special Tests	Not applicable
Referral/ Diagnostic Procedure	Refer to a pulmonary physician. Chest x-ray; CBC; sputum cultures.
Classification of Injury	Not applicable

Medical Term	Rhinitis
Common Term	Cold
Mechanisms	Viral infection that affects the mucus membranes of the respiratory system, causing inflammation and mucus secretion. Muscle inflammation is also common.
Symptoms	Sore throat; runny nose and/or congestion; possibly aching muscles.
Signs	Clear or colored nasal discharge; fever; posterior pharynx injection; possible anterior cervical lymphadenopathy.
Special Tests	Not applicable
Referral/ Diagnostic Procedure	Refer to a physician. CBC and/or strep screen in unclear cases.
Classification of Injury	Not applicable

Medical Term	Rhinitis, allergic
Common Term	Hay fever
Mechanisms	Allergic reaction to dust, pollen, or chemicals, leading to an overreaction of the body's immune system.
Symptoms	Headache; runny nose; fatigue; watery eyes; itchy nose and eyes; sometimes head stuffiness and sore throat.
Signs	Clear watery discharge from the eyes and nose; "allergic shadows" underneath the eyes; injection of the posterior pharynx; sometimes hoarseness.
Special Tests	Not applicable
Referral/ Diagnostic Procedure	Refer to a physician with expertise in allergies. Allergy testing can be done in those individuals who have severe disease, but most patients are treated empirically.
Classification of Injury	Not applicable

Medical Term	Rubella
Common Term	German measles
Mechanisms	Infection with rubella virus.
Symptoms	Rash; drowsiness.
Signs	Low-grade fever with tender occipital, postcervical, and postauricular adenopathy and a salmon-colored discrete rash spreading from the head and neck to the rest of the body within 1 day.
Special Tests	Not applicable
Referral/ Diagnostic Procedure	Refer to a physician.
Classification of Injury	Not applicable

Medical Term	**Rubeola**
Common Term	Measles
Mechanisms	Infection with rubeola virus.
Symptoms	Cough; coryza; photophobia.
Signs	Fever; conjunctivitis; violaceous, confluent lesions, beginning at the face and neck, then spreading to the trunk and extremities. The patient may be very ill.
Special Tests	Not applicable
Referral/ Diagnostic Procedure	Refer to a physician.
Classification of Injury	Not applicable

Medical Term	Sickle cell anemia
Common Term	Same as above
Mechanisms	A genetic abnormality in hemoglobin, occurring in almost exclusively in the African-American population, which leads to red blood cells that become sickle-shaped. These "sickled" cells cause occlusion of small blood vessels, which are experienced as sickle cell crises by the patient.
Symptoms	Intermittent episodes of severe pain at various locations of the body; possible leg pain.
Signs	Obvious distress; possible jaundice; sometimes skin or pulmonary infections.
Special Tests	Not applicable
Referral/ Diagnostic Procedure	Refer to a physician. Sickle cell screen; hemoglobin electrophoresis; CBC.
Classification of Injury	Not applicable

Medical Term	**Sinusitis**
Common Term	Sinus infection
Mechanisms	Bacterial or viral infection of the sinus cavities, of which there are three principal pairs: the ethmoid, the maxillary, and the frontal.
Symptoms	Headache; stuffiness; postnasal drainage; sore throat; a feeling of pressure in the affected sinuses.
Signs	Tenderness to percussion over the affected sinuses; injection of the posterior pharynx; fever; colored nasal discharge.
Special Tests	Not applicable
Referral/ Diagnostic Procedure	Refer to a physician. Sometimes sinus x-rays are done, but patients are usually treated empirically.
Classification of Injury	Not applicable

Medical Term	**Tinea versicolor**
Common Term	Yeast infection
Mechanisms	Fungal infection
Symptoms	Pain and itching when the body is overheated.
Signs	Black skin appears as white or pink areas; light skin appears as dark, white, or pink areas. This condition is often more visible in summer, due to lack of tanning on affected areas. It is found on the chest, neck, and abdomen.
Special Tests	Not applicable
Referral/ Diagnostic Procedure	Refer to a physician.
Classification of Injury	Not applicable

Medical Term	Tetanus
Common Term	Lockjaw
Mechanisms	Infection by *Clostridium tetani*, a bacteria that is found in soil contaminated by animal manure. The organism enters the body through a contaminated wound and eventually enters the central nervous system.
Symptoms	Pain at the site of wound or puncture, followed by hypertonicity and spasm of regional muscles. Characteristic difficulty in opening the mouth is usually apparent within 48 hours.
Signs	Recurrent spasm of the regional muscle groups; obvious anxiety and irritability. Fever in severe cases.
Special Tests	Not applicable
Referral/ Diagnostic Procedure	Refer to a physician. Tetanus shot.
Classification of Injury	Not applicable

Medical Term	Tonsillitis
Common Term	Sore throat
Mechanisms	Viral or bacterial infection of tonsils.
Symptoms	Sore throat; chills; lethargy; sometimes headache.
Signs	Tonsils reddened and swollen; pus sometimes present; anterior cervical lymphadenopathy.
Special Tests	Not applicable
Referral/ Diagnostic Procedure	Refer to a physician. Strep screen and mononucleosis screen.
Classification of Injury	Not applicable

Medical Term	**Upper respiratory infection**
Common Term	Common cold
Mechanisms	Viral infection of upper respiratory system, including the head and throat. Mycoplasma is an important nonviral cause of upper respiratory infections.
Symptoms	Coryza; nasal stuffiness; sore throat.
Signs	Nasal discharge; postnasal drip; sometimes fever.
Special Tests	Not applicable
Referral/ Diagnostic Procedure	Refer to a physician.
Classification of Injury	Not applicable

Medical Term	**Urethritis**
Common Term	Same as above
Mechanisms	Inflammation of urethra secondary to infection or irritative agents.
Symptoms	Burning and discomfort on urination. Sometimes urethral discharge is noted.
Signs	None unless discharge is present.
Special Tests	Not applicable
Referral/ Diagnostic Procedure	Refer to a urologist. Urinalysis and urethral culture.
Classification of Injury	Not applicable

Medical Term	**Urinary tract infection**
Common Term	Kidney/bladder infection
Mechanisms	Bacterial infection.
Symptoms	Painful urination (dysuria), frequency, urgency; sometimes flank pain and nausea or vomiting.
Signs	Suprapubic tenderness; costovertebral angle (midback) tenderness; fever with kidney involvement.
Special Tests	Not applicable
Referral/ Diagnostic Procedure	Refer to a urologist. Urinalysis; CBC in severe cases.
Classification of Injury	Not applicable

Medical Term	Vaginitis
Common Term	Same as above
Mechanisms	Yeast, bacterial, or trichomonas infection.
Symptoms	Itching; pain; colored and/or "cottage cheese" discharge; painful sexual intercourse.
Signs	Colored, sometimes malodorous, discharge with inflammation of vaginal mucosa.
Special Tests	Not applicable
Referral/ Diagnostic Procedure	Refer to a gynecologist. Wet mount and potassium hydroxide prep.
Classification of Injury	Not applicable

Medical Term	Varicella
Common Term	Chicken pox
Mechanisms	Viral infection that affects the skin and mucus membranes, but which in more severe cases may affect other body systems such as the lungs.
Symptoms	Itchy lesions scattered over the body, sometimes accompanied by malaise and headache.
Signs	"Dewdrop on rose" lesion, which appears as a small clear blister on a red background. These lesions appear at differing times, so that some are crusting over while others are still appearing.
Special Tests	Not applicable
Referral/ Diagnostic Procedure	Refer to a physician.
Classification of Injury	Not applicable

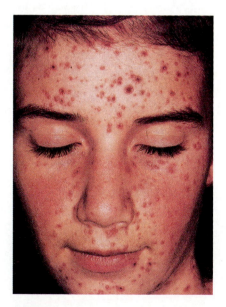

Chicken pox.

Medical Term	**Viral hepatitis**
Common Term	Same as above
Mechanisms	Viral infection of liver, leading to destruction of liver cells and, in extreme cases, death.
Symptoms	Nausea; vomiting; malaise; weakness; loss of appetite; right upper quadrant discomfort.
Signs	Dark urine; low-grade fever; tender right upper quadrant; obvious illness; in advanced cases, jaundice.
Special Tests	Not applicable
Referral/ Diagnostic Procedure	Refer to physician with expertise in infectious disease. Blood tests for type of infectious hepatitis.
Classification of Injury	Not applicable

INITIAL MANAGEMENT OF ATHLETIC INJURIES

Chapter 21

This chapter presents various aspects of the initial management of athletic injuries. Basic guidelines for administering treatment are presented, and the physiologic effects of the treatment modality are examined. The manner in which the body responds to injury is presented and acts as the foundation on which the rationale for the use of ice is established.

While it is critical that the athletic trainer know proper treatment protocol, such knowledge alone is not an adequate foundation on which to build the clinical skills of the athletic trainer. It is crucial that athletic trainers know the exact reason any modality is applied, as well as the specific effects that the modality has on the area being treated. For that reason the discussion of initial treatment will begin with the response of the injured tissue to the actual injury.

The Inflammatory Response

The immediate result of the injurious episode is the damage realized by the tissue. Depending on its type, tissue may be strained, sprained, fractured, or otherwise damaged. Regardless of the cause, certain events occur within the tissue as an immediate response to the injury episode. This is commonly referred to as primary injury,[1] which is any tissue damage directly resulting from the force or agent that caused the injury.

Inflammation is defined as the body's nonspecific response to irritation or injury. The first event occurring during the inflammatory response is vasoconstriction, followed within minutes by vasodilation.[2] Vasodilation allows more blood flow to the injured area, which will increase the amount of swelling. Chemicals such as bradykinin and histamine are released into the area, which further increases swelling and tissue sensitivity. These vascular, cellular, and chemical events collectively cause the traditional signs of inflammation: heat, redness, swelling, and pain.

In addition to the initial tissue damage experienced at the immediate time of injury, more tissue damage may result from secondary hypoxia.[1,2] If enough swelling has occurred, blood supply to the injured area may be impeded. Secondary hypoxia is the result of compromised blood flow, and therefore less oxygen, to the damaged tissue. Deprived of oxygen, more tissue is damaged than was originally from the initial injury.

Rationale for ICE

With a basic understanding of how tissue responds to injury it is possible to formulate a treatment plan. Acute injuries should be treated with cold application, compression, and elevation. The acronym *ICE* is commonly used by athletic trainers in reference to the initial treatment of injuries.

   I — ice or cold application
   C — compression applied to the injured area
   E — elevation of the injured body part

Cold application will not decrease the severity of the initial injury but it will assist in decreasing the amount of tissue damaged as the result of secondary hypoxia. The most significant impact of cold application is decreased tissue temperature.[3] Decreasing tissue temperature causes vasoconstriction, thereby decreasing the degree to which swelling is present and is allowed to compromise oxygen to the tissue. Decreased tissue temperature also slows nerve conduction velocity, which decreases the amount of pain experienced by the athlete. Muscle spasm is reduced by decreasing muscle spindle firing. The rate of release of bradykinin, histamine, and prostaglandin are slowed, resulting in less pain and swelling. As tissue temperature decreases, cell metabolism decreases correspondingly. Slowing the metabolic rate allows cells in the injured area to be sustained with less oxygen than normal. This is beneficial because less tissue death will result from secondary hypoxia.

During cold application, a phenomena commonly called the *hunting reaction* will occur.[3,5] This reaction is simply a protective mechanism initiated by the body in response to decreased tissue temperature. As cooled blood is transported out of the injured area, the body responds as if there is an urgent need to elevate tissue temperature. This is most likely an attempt by the body to protect itself from tissue damage caused by frostbite.

Rationale for Compression

The use of compression during the initial treatment of acute athletic injuries is more closely related to swelling control than is the use of ice.[4] Whether ice alone or ice with compression promotes a greater decrease in tissue temperature or deeper tissue cooling is not known. Unlike ice, external compression has no demonstrable effect on cell metabolism. While there is no clearly established link between compression and tissue temperature decrease, it is still recommended on the basis of the effect of external compression on edema. External compression, alone or with ice, has been proven effective in reducing edema.[3] External compression acts to slow the escape of fluid from damaged tissue.

Elevation of the injured limb or area helps reduce the amount of swelling. Gravity causes more blood to pool in the extremities. Elevating the limb eliminates the effects of gravity. Elevation also facilitates venous return from the injured area. Care should be exercised to ensure that the limb or injured area is not in a gravity-dependent position during treatment.

Application Techniques

The most appropriate method for application of ice will vary, depending on the injured area. Regardless of the technique used, certain precautions should be taken. The athlete should be informed that he or she will experience a sequence of sensations as the treatment progresses. Initially the athlete will experience a cold sensation. This feeling of intense cold will be followed by a stinging sensation. A burning or aching feeling will be felt next, followed ultimately by numbness.

Although it is relatively uncommon, some athletes will exhibit an allergic reaction to ice treatment. In such cases the athlete may have a welt on the skin where the ice was applied. If an athlete displays such a reaction, the use of ice is contraindicated.

Any one of a variety of techniques may be used during the application of ice. The initial treatment of an injury dictates which method is the treatment of choice. The method used should allow the incorporation of both compression and elevation. This being the case, selecting a cold whirlpool for the initial treatment is not appropriate, as it allows neither compression or elevation. A similar situation exists with ice massage. While ice massage is a valuable treatment in other situations, it is not the appropriate treatment for an initial injury.

Ice Packs

Research has established[3,5] that ice packs applied directly to the skin will not cause frostbite. Research done by Knight[3] indicates that ice applied directly to the skin is much more effective than ice placed over a towel or elastic wrap. The best method of application is directly to the skin.

The duration of ice application should be at least 20 minutes for the initial treatment. The treatment may be extended to as long as 30 minutes to be more effective. The longer period allows the body to pass through the vasodilation response caused by the cold and enter into a second phase of vasoconstriction.[3]

The type of ice that is applied may influence the effectiveness of the treatment. Crushed ice is preferred because it will allow the pack to conform better to the shape of the area or body part being treated.[5]

Commercial Cold Packs

Unlike ice packs, commercial cold packs should not be applied directly to the skin. The pack should be wrapped in a wet towel and then applied to the area being treated.[5] A benefit of commercial cold packs is the ability of the pack to conform to the body. A commercial cold pack is more comfortable than an ice pack when placed beneath a pneumatic intermittent compression sleeve.

Treatment time when using a commercial cold pack is 20 minutes. The pack may be applied for 20 minutes and then removed for 20 minutes. This cycle should be repeated for 2 hours.[5] It is important to place the limb or area in an elevated position during the treatment.

References

1. Arnheim DD and Prentice WE: *Principles of athletic training*, ed 8, ,St. Louis, 1993, Mosby.
2. Caillet R: *Soft tissue pain and disability*, Philadelphia, 1988, F.A. Davis.
3. Knight KL: *Cryotherapy: theory, technique, and physiology*, Chattanooga, Tenn., 1985, Chattanooga Corp.
4. Merrick MA et al: The effect of ice and compression wraps on intramuscular temperatures at various depths, *J Athlet Train*, 28(3):236-245, 1993.
5. Prentice WE: *Therapeutic modalities in sports medicine*, ed 2, St. Louis, 1990, Mosby.

■ APPENDIX OF MEDICAL SPECIALTIES ■

Allergist

Physician whose specialty pertains to the study of the human body's reaction to foreign substances.

Anesthesiologist

Physician who manages the procedures for rendering a patient insensible to pain during surgical procedures and for the patient's life support during and after surgery.

Cardiologist

Physician whose specialty pertains to caring for defects and diseases of the cardiovascular system.

Dentist

Person who practices the care of the teeth and associated structures, including prevention, diagnosis, and treatment of diseases of the teeth and gums.

Dermatologist

Physician who deals with the medical aspects of skin disorders and diseases.

Emergency medicine physician

Physician whose medical practice emphasizes the prehospital care and the acute care of other specialities of medicine.

Endocrinologist

Physician who deals with the diagnosis and treatment of the hormone-producing glandular and metabolic systems.

Family practice physician

Provider of primary health care to the whole family through a coordinated plan with other specialized physicians and community services.

Gastroenterologist

Physician whose practice pertains to a subspecialty of internal medicine dealing with the diagnosis and treatment of diseases and disorders of the digestive system.

Gynecologist

Physician whose practice pertains to the care of disorders and diseases of the female reproductive tract.

Hematologist

Physician whose practice pertains to the diagnosis and treatment of blood disorders.

Infectious diseases physician

Physician whose practice deals with the diagnosis and treatment of communicable and contagious diseases.

Internist

Physician who provides primary care to adults full time and treats diseases of the internal organs by other than surgical means.

Medical oncologist

Physician whose practice pertains to the diagnosis and treatment of neoplastic diseases (i.e., cancer).

Nephrologist

Physician whose practice pertains to the treatment and diagnosis of renal (kidney) diseases and other related problems of the patient.

Neurologic surgeon

Physician who deals with the central, peripheral, and autonomic nervous system and covers diagnosis and, often, surgery.

Neurologist

Physician whose practice pertains to the diagnosis and treatment of disorders of the nervous system.

Nuclear medicine

Branch of medicine that does diagnostic work using radioactive isotopes and larger amounts for the treatment of diseases.

Obstetrician

Physician whose practice pertains to the care of a woman before, during, and after her pregnancy.

Ophthalmologist

Physician whose practice is concerned with the function, diseases, and abnormalities of the eye.

Orthodontist

Dentist who deals with the prevention and correction of abnormalities or misalignment of teeth.

Orthopedic Surgeon

Surgeon whose practice pertains to the restoration of normal function to a deformed, diseased, or injured part of the musculoskeletal system using medical, surgical, and physical rehabilitation means.

Otolaryngologist

Surgeon (head and neck surgeon) who deals with all diseases and lesions above the clavicle, except for visual and eye-related diseases and lesions of the brain.

Otorhinolaryngologist

Physician who deals with the science of the ear, nose, and larynx and their function and diseases.

Pathologist

Physician whose practice pertains to a branch of medicine concerned with the cause, manifestation, diagnosis, and outcome of diseases.

Pediatrician

Physician whose practice pertains to the care of young people from birth to adolescence with concern for their physical, mental, and emotional health.

Pedodontist

Dentist who cares for the teeth of children.

Periodonist

Person who practices in the field of dentistry dealing with treatment of diseases of the tissues around the teeth.

Physiatrist (physical medicine)

Physician whose medical practice is concerned with the diagnosis of the disease process underlying the disability, but with a focus on the functional disability and its management for wellness.

Plastic surgeon

Surgeon whose specialty deals with the repair and correction of congential defects, trauma, and cancer reconstruction.

Proctologist

Physician whose specialty pertains to the treatment and surgery of the colon and rectum.

Prosthodontist

Dentist who specializes in fixed and removable false teeth (such as dentures, crowns, bridges).

Psychiatrist

Physician whose practice of medicine deals with the mental and emotional disorders of the patient.

Pulmonologist

Physician who diagnoses and treats diseases of the respiratory system.

Radiologist

1) Diagnostic: Physician who uses the application of x-rays and other forms of radiant energy to diagnose disease. 2) Therapeutic: physician who specializes in the treatment of the patient with x-rays, radium, and radionuclides.

Rheumatologist

Physician whose practice pertains to the diagnosis and treatment of rheumatic diseases and musculoskeletal problems.

Thoracic surgeon

Surgeon whose specialty deals with the chest cavity containing the heart, lungs, and esophagus.

Urologist

Physician whose practice pertains to a surgical subspeciality concerned with the medical and surgical treatment of disorders and diseases of the female urinary tract and male urogenital tract.

■ BIBLIOGRAPHY ■

Arnheim DD: *Essentials in athletic training*, ed 3, St Louis, 1995, Mosby.

Arnheim DD, Prentice WE: *Principles of athletic training*, ed 8, St Louis, 1993, Mosby.

Berkow R and others: *The Merck manual of diagnosis and therapy*, ed 13, Rahway, NJ, 1977, Merck Sharp and Dohme Research Laboratories.

Booher JM, Thibodeau GA: *Athletic injury assessment*, ed 3, St Louis, 1994, Mosby.

Curwin S, Stanish WD: *Tendinitis: its etiology and treatment*, Lexington, MA, 1984, DC Heath.

Dayton OW: *Athletic training and conditioning*, New York, 1965, Ronald Press.

Ellison AE and others: *Athletic training and sports medicine*, Chicago, 1984, American Academy of Orthopedic Surgeons.

Evans RC: *Illustrated essentials in orthopedic physical assessment*, St Louis, 1994, Mosby.

Fahey TD: *Athletic training: principles and practice*, Palo Alto, CA, 1986, Mayfield Publishing.

Habif TP: *Clinical dermatology: a color guide to diagnosis and therapy*, ed 2, St Louis, 1990, Mosby.

Hartley A: *Practical joint assessment: a sports medicine manual*, St. Louis, 1990, Mosby.

Hay WW, Jr, Groothuis JR, Hayward AR, and Levin MI, editors: *Current pediatric diagnosis and treatment*, Norwalk, CT, 1995, Appleton & Lange.

Hirata I: *The doctor and the athlete*, Philadelphia, 1974, JB Lippincott.

Kulund DN: *The injured athlete*, Philadelphia, 1982, JB Lippincott.

Magee DJ: *Orthopedic physical assessment*, ed 2, Philadelphia, 1992, WB Saunders.

Nicholas JA, Hershman EB: *The upper extremity in sports medicine*, St Louis, 1990, Mosby.

O'Donoghue DH: *Treatment of injuries to athletes*, ed 3, Philadelphia, 1976, WB Saunders.

Rachum A and others: *Standard nomenclature of athletic injuries*, Chicago, 1968, American Medical Association.

Ragge NK, Eastly DL: *Immediate eye care: an illustrated manual*, St Louis, 1990, Mosby.

Rawlinson K: *Athletic training*, North Palm Beach, FL, 1980, The Athletic Institute.

Read M: *Sports Injuries*, New York, 1984, Arco Publishing.

Rosen P and others: *Diagnostic radiology in emergency medicine*, St Louis, 1992, Mosby.

Roy S, Irvin R: *Sports medicine: prevention, evaluation, management, and rehabilitation*, Englewood Cliffs, NJ, 1983, Prentice-Hall.

Taylor AD: *How to choose a medical specialty*, ed 2, Philadelphia, 1993, WB Saunders.

Thomas CL, editor: *Taber's cyclopedic medical dictionary*, ed 13, Philadelphia, 1973, FA Davis.

Williams JGP: *Color atlas of injury in sport*, St Louis, 1980, Mosby.

■ PHOTO CREDITS ■

Chapter 2

pp. 29, 30b, 31b, 32, 33b, 34, Rosen/Doris/ Barkin/Barkin/Markovchick: *Diagnostic radiology in emergency medicine*, ed 1, St. Louis, 1992, Mosby.

Chapter 3

pp. 43, 45, 47, McDonald/Avery: *Dentistry for the child and adolescent*, ed 6, St. Louis, 1990, Mosby; pp. 50a & b, 51, 52, 53a & b, 55a, 56, 57, 64a & b, Ragge/Easty: *Immediate eye care*, ed 1, St. Louis, 1990, Mosby; pp. 54, 65, Williams: *Color atlas of injury in sport*, ed 2, St. Louis, 1990, Mosby; p. 67, Booher/Thibodeau: *Athletic Injury Assessment*, ed 3, St. Louis, 1994, Mosby; p. 70, redrawn from Arnheim/Prentice: *Principles of athletic training*, ed 8, St. Louis, 1993, Mosby

Chapter 4

p. 85, 86, Rosen/Doris/Barkin/Barkin/Markovchick: *Diagnostic radiology in emergency medicine*, ed 1, St. Louis, 1992, Mosby; p. 87, 89, Nicholas/Hershman: *The lower extremity and spine in sports medicine*, ed 2, St. Louis, 1995, Mosby; pp. 88, 94, Williams: *Color atlas of injury in sport*, ed 2, St. Louis, 1990, Mosby.

Chapter 5

p.106, Booher/Thibodeau: *Athletic injury assessment*, ed 3, St. Louis, 1994, Mosby; p. 108a & b, redrawn from Arnheim/Prentice: *Principles of athletic training*, ed 8, St. Louis, 1993, Mosby; p. 109, 113a & b, 115, Rosen/ Doris/Barkin/Barkin/Markovchick: *Diagnostic radiology in emergency medicine*, ed 1, St. Louis, 1992, Mosby; p. 110, 117a & b, 123, Nicholas/Hershman: *The lower extremity and spine in sports medicine*, ed 2, St. Louis, 1990, Mosby; p. 112a & b, 121a & b, Williams: *Color atlas of injury in sport*, ed 2, St. Louis, 1990, Mosby.

Chapter 6

pp.135, 139, Williams: *Color atlas of injury in sport*, ed 2, St. Louis, 1990, Mosby; p. 137, Nicholas/Hershman: *The lower extremity and spine in sports medicine*, ed 2, St. Louis, 1990, Mosby.

Chapter 7

pp. 145, 146, redrawn from Arnheim/Prentice: *Principles of athletic training*, ed 8, St. Louis, 1993, Mosby; pp. 149, 160a & b, Nicholas/ Hershman: *The lower extremity and spine in sports medicine*, ed 2, St. Louis, 1990, Mosby; pp. 152, 161a & b, Williams: *Color atlas of injury in sport*, ed 2, St. Louis, 1990, Mosby.

Chapter 8

pp. 170, 171, 172, Rosen/Doris/Barkin/ Barkin/Markovchick: *Diagnostic radiology in emergency medicine*, ed 1, St. Louis, 1992, Mosby; p. 175, Booher/Thibodeau: *Athletic injury assessment*, ed 3, St. Louis, 1994, Mosby; p. 176, Nicholas/Hershman: *The lower extremity and spine in sports medicine*, ed 2, St. Louis, 1995, Mosby.

Chapter 9

pp. 193, 201, 207a & b, Nicholas/Hershman: *The lower extremity and spine in sports medicine*, ed 2, St. Louis, 1995, Mosby; pp. 194, 199, Rosen/Doris/Barkin/Barkin/Markovchick: *Diagnostic radiology in emergency medicine*, ed 1, St. Louis, 1992, Mosby; p. 203, Booher/ Thibodeau: *Athletic injury assessment*, ed 3, St. Louis, 1994, Mosby.

Chapter 10

pp. 220, 221, 223, 224, Rosen/Doris/Barkin/ Barkin/Markovchick: *Diagnostic radiology in emergency medicine*, ed 1, St. Louis, 1992, Mosby.

Chapter 11

pp. 226, 231, 234, Rosen/Doris/Barkin/Barkin/Markovchick: *Diagnostic radiology in emergency medicine*, ed 1, St. Louis, 1992, Mosby.

Chapter 12

pp. 249, 251, 258, Rosen/Doris/Barkin/Barkin/Markovchick: *Diagnostic radiology in emergency medicine*, ed 1, St. Louis, 1992, Mosby.

Chapter 13

pp. 269, 275, Rosen/Doris/Barkin/Barkin/
Markovchick: *Diagnostic radiology in emergency
medicine*, ed 1, St. Louis, 1992, Mosby.

Chapter 14

pp. 284, 287, redrawn from Arnheim/Prentice:
Principles of athletic training, ed 8, St. Louis,
1993, Mosby.

Chapter 15

pp. 300a & b, 301, 310, 317, 319, redrawn
from Arnheim/Prentice: *Principles of athletic
training*, ed 8, St. Louis, 1993, Mosby; p. 308,
Booher/Thibodeau: *Athletic injury assessment*,
ed 3, St. Louis, 1994, Mosby; p. 313, Williams:
Color atlas of injury in sport, ed 2, St. Louis,
1990, Mosby.

Chapter 16

pp. 344, 355, 358, redrawn from Arnheim/
Prentice: *Principles of athletic training*, ed 8,
St. Louis, 1993, Mosby; p. 356, Williams: *Color
atlas of injury in sport*, ed 2, St. Louis, 1990,
Mosby

Chapter 17

p. 366, Rosen/Doris/Barkin/Barkin/Markov-
chick: *Diagnostic radiology in emergency medicine*, ed 1, St. Louis, 1992, Mosby; p. 374,
redrawn from Arnheim/Prentice: *Principles of
athletic training*, ed 8, St. Louis, 1993, Mosby.

Chapter 18

pp. 394, 397, Rosen/Doris/Barkin/Barkin/
Markovchick: *Diagnostic radiology in emergency
medicine*, ed 1, St. Louis, 1992, Mosby; pp.
404, 410, redrawn from Arnheim/Prentice:
Principles of athletic training, ed 8, St. Louis,
1993, Mosby.

Chapter 19

pp. 422, 424, 427, 428, 429, 431, 433, 434, 435,
436, 437, 438, 439, 440, 441, 443, 444, 445, 446,
447, Habif: *Clinical dermatology*, ed 2, St. Louis,
1990, Mosby; p. 430, Vallotton/Dubas: *Color
atlas of mountain medicine*, ed 1, St. Louis, 1992,
Mosby; p. 442, Williams: *Color atlas of injury in
sport*, ed 2, St. Louis, 1990, Mosby.

■ INDEX ■

Supination, 10
Suprapatellar bursitis, 303
Sweating, 432
Swimmer's ear, 72
Swimmer's shoulder, 111
Symptom, definition of, 12
Syncope, 10
Synovitis, 10
  of hip, 281

T

Tachycardia, 10
Tachypnea, 10
Tackler's exostosis, 135
Talar tilt test, ankle injury and, 380
Tarsal fracture, 397
Tarsal tunnel syndrome, 415
Temporomandibular dysfunction, 78
Temporomandibular joint luxation, 71
Tendinitis, 10, 16, 300
  joint range of motion and, 97
Tendon, 10
  achilles, rupture of, 363
Tennis elbow, 145, 146
Tennis leg, 357
Tenosynovitis, 10, 17, 124, 205
  joint range of motion and, 97
Tension pneumothorax, 224
Testicle, 10
Tetanus, 494
Theca, 10
Thigh contusion, 288
Thigh injury, 285-300
Thomas test, hip flexion contracture
  and, 284
Thoracic arm injury, 211-224
Thoracic outlet syndrome, tests and,
  129
Throat contusion, 84
Throat infection, 485
Thrower's shoulder, 111
Thyroid cartilage, fracture of, 85
Tibia
  chondral fracture of, 369
  fracture of, 354
  osteochondral fracture of, 369
  plateau fracture of, 355
  stress fracture of, 353
Tibiofemoral luxation, 308
Tinea corporis, 443
Tinea cruris, 444
Tinea pedis, 445
Tinea versicolor, 493
Tinel's sign, carpal tunnel syndrome
  and, 183
Tinnitus, 10
Tongue laceration, 69
Tonsillitis, 495

Tooth
  abscess of, 43
  avulsed, 44
  caries and, 45
  fracture of, 46
  intrusion of, 48
  luxation of, 49
Torn cartilage, 312
Torticollis, 94
Transient paralysis, 8
Transient quadriplegia, 90
Transverse process fracture, 229
Trauma, 10
Traumatic arthritis, 3
Traumatic tunica vaginalis hydrocele,
  474
Trendelenburg test, gluteus medius
  muscle and, 284
Triceps strain, 138
Trichomonas, 10
Trigeminal nerve, 36-37
Trochanteric bursitis, 266
Trochlear nerve, 36
Turf toe, 414

U

Ulcer, 11
Ulna
  epiphyseal plate injury of, 176
  fracture of, 153
Ulnar collateral ligament of the
  thumb sprain, 203
Ulnar nerve, 11
  contusion of, 156
  injury of, 159
  nerve distribution test and, 163-164
  test, 208
Ulnar neuropathy, 206
Unconsciousness, 11
Unguis incarnates, 416
Upper arm injury, 131-139
Upper respiratory infection, 496
Urethritis, 497
Urinary tract infection, 498
Urticaria, 446

V

Vaginitis, 499
Vagus nerve, 37
Valgus, 11
Valgus (abduction) stress test, knee
  injury and, 339, 340
Valgus and varus stress test, flexor
  digitorum profundus tendon
  rupture and, 208
Valsalva test, 95
  intrathecal pressure and, 241
Varicella, 500

Varus, 11
Varus (adduction) stress test, knee
  injury and, 339
Vascular occlusion, wrist injury and,
  183
Venereal disease, 458, 469
Venereal wart, 461
Verruca plantaris, 417
Verruca vulgaris, 447
Vesicle, 11
Viral hepatitis, 501
Virus, 11
Volar, definition of, 11
Volar plate injury, 207
Volkmann's contracture, 162
Vomiting, 11

W

Wart, 447
Water on the knee, 322
Well leg/straight leg raise test, 240
Wens, 445
Whiplash injury, 92
Wind knocked out, 215
Winging scapula, 107
Wound, definition of, 22
Wrist contusion, 174
Wrist extension test, lateral
  epicondylitis and, 163
Wrist ganglion, 173
Wrist, injury of, 167-183
  Allen's test and, 183
  evaluation tests and, 182-183
  flexion of, medial epicondylitis
    and, 163
  luxation of, 179
  pronation of, medial epicondylitis,
    163
  sprain of, 180
    range of motion and, 182
  strain of, 181
    range of motion and, 182
  tendinitis of, range of motion and,
    182
  tenosynovitis of, 191
  range of motion and, 182
  vascular occlusion and, 183
Wryneck, 94

Y

Yeast infection, 493
Yergason test, biceps tendon and, 128